Break Free From Atrial Fibrillation

And Take Your Life Back

LEONARD JENSEN

Table of Contents

INTRODUCTION – PART 1

The thought of sleeping and not waking up the next day is perhaps your greatest fear. Or you're damn scared you are going to lose one of your loved ones and relatives to the cold fists of death. Like everyone, you must have thought that cancer is the deadliest of all diseases and infections. But what happens at that moment when your heart suddenly begins to pound away speedily like a bolt of lightning striking across the gray lines of the sky? That moment perhaps is the scariest moment of your life.

You are caught in a state of dilemma, whether what you are feeling and experiencing is true or not. You begin to wonder if your heart is playing tricks on you. Your heartbeat rate, rather than reduce, continues to increase drastically. From a hundred and twenty beats per minute, the figure soars to a hundred and fifty. Still, it does not stop there. It continues until it reaches as high as a hundred and eighty. At this point, the rate at which your heart is beating is two or three times the rate at which it should be.

Reality hits you most unexpectedly. What you have heard several times in the news being discussed by experts, to which you paid little or no attention to, is now happening to you. Your life, your health, your heart, which you have treated with little concern your whole life, become the most important things to you at that moment. The pounding and the vibrations are loud and clear enough for your ears to decipher. You experience some pain in your chest region. All other thoughts: the thoughts of the clothes you were going to wear, the food you were going to eat, the party you were going to attend with your friends and colleagues at work, the preparations for Christmas, the all-ladies or all-guys reunion you planned to hold; disappear from your mind immediately. The thought of whether you will make it out alive or answer the call to heaven rings a bell in your mind.

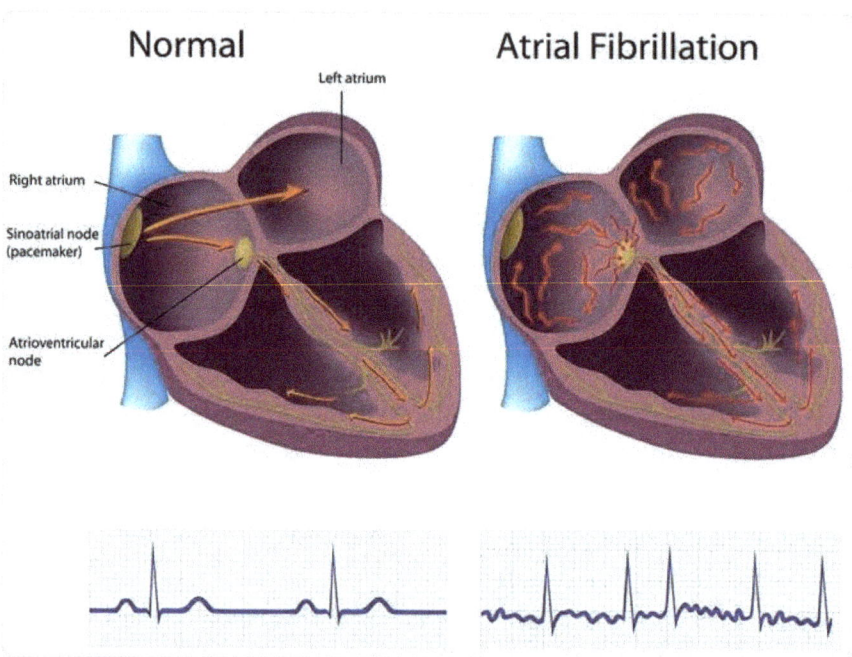

If you were standing when you had the attack, you unconsciously choose to sit down, and if you were sitting down, you would want to lie down flat on the bed. No other thing is right there in your mind but death. As the heartbeats continue rapidly, another thought rears its ugly presence in your mind. The idea of having a heart attack screams loud in your head.

If you are such a person who prays when confronted with challenges or health issues, you begin to pray and ask for wellness. Even if you are not the praying type, you probably will resort to begging God at this moment because it seems like the perfect thing to do.

If the symptoms, instead of reducing, continue to rise, you think of another alternative. You pick up your phone and try to reach out to your doctor. If he is not reachable, you go ahead and dial 911. Your hands are shaking conspicuously and your mind is unable to think straight. The process of collecting your details and information, such as your name, address, and your exact location in your home by the dispatcher, can be pretty difficult.

You are asked if you could make it to the front door of your house. If you have the strength, you give it a go. Like watching a movie at the cinema, everything seems to be occurring in slow motion. You feel like the world is at a standstill.

And when you finally make it to the door, all your strength and energy vanish. You slump to the floor at this moment and wait patiently for help to arrive.

If you or a relative have ever had this experience at any point in your life, you should know that you are not alone. What you have gone through is known as Atrial Fibrillation. Myriads of people across all regions of the world have, at one point or another, have had this experience. If they haven't, they must have come across someone who had had it or better still heard someone recount his knowledge about it.

Having said that, many people still do not know much about this medical condition.

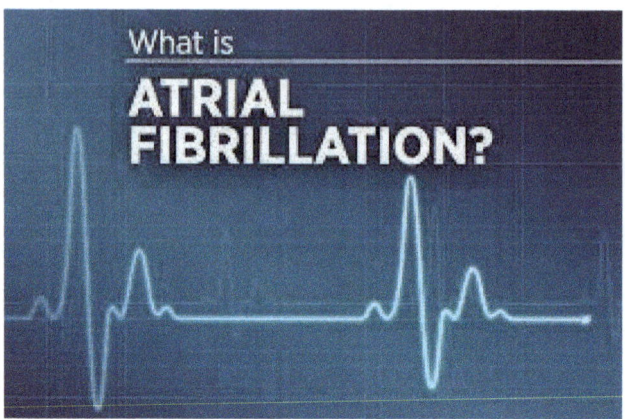

The big question now is what is Atrial Fibrillation?

Atrial Fibrillation, mainly referred to as AFIB, is a health condition involving an unpredictable and uncontrollable episode of destructive electrical activities in the heart's upper chambers. In most cases, it results in irregular and rapid heartbeats that deteriorate as time passes by if not well managed and treated. This health condition is said to be the most frequently diagnosed arrhythmia in the world. You probably haven't heard that word before, have you? And if you have, probably I should remind you of the meaning. Arrhythmia is a health condition characterized by irregularity and abnormality in the rate at which the heart beats.

If you have or know someone who has had experienced this medical condition, the good news is that you are not alone. A lot of people across the world have suffered the same fate as you. So, there is no need to be scared. Former presidents of the United States of

America, Richard Nixon and George H.W Bush, both suffered it. Also, former vice presidents Dick Cheney and Joe Biden had it. World renowned and famous singers such as Elton John and Barry Manilow suffered this health condition. So have comedians such as Howie Mandel and Ellen DeGeneres. Even basketballers who have earned themselves a name in the Basketball Hall of Fame like Bill Bradly and Larry Bird had experienced it. The list of casualties doesn't stop here.

Reports have shown that one out of every four American adults will have atrial fibrillation to contend with at some point in their lives. Studies have also suggested that for some groups of people residing in the United States, the chances of suffering atrial fibrillation may be as high as one out of every three. Research has also established that more than sixty million residents of the United States have the risk of suffering at least one episode of atrial fibrillation in their lives. Taking a closer look at the global scenes, with the rising population of aged people, the incidence of atrial fibrillation appears to be on the rise. Globally, statistics have it that more than sixty-five million people above the age of thirty-five have been diagnosed with atrial fibrillation. Beyond the reports and facts, thousands of millions of people across the world have not been diagnosed yet.

When you suffer from atrial fibrillation, you are not suffering from it alone. Your family, parents, children, siblings, friends, and relatives suffer with you. Since the average amount for treating this medical condition hovers around 20,000 USSD (the cost might be more than this in some cases), even lucky people who have no personal experience with atrial fibrillation are indirectly affected. That is due to high rates of insurance that support those in the pool or high taxes to lend help to those who are not insured, underinsured, or insured via government programs. Also, it is excluding the cost and amount spent on lost productivity.

If you have chosen to read the content of this book, there is a high chance that you have had an experience like the one illustrated in the previous paragraphs, or you know a person who has. This piece focuses on curing atrial fibrillation. So, sit back and enjoy.

CHAPTER ONE: THE STORY BEHIND ATRIAL FIBRILLATION (AFIB)

When Mike was diagnosed with atrial fibrillation, his doctor frankly confessed that there wasn't anything he could do about it. It occurred in the late 1990s.

"Whether you believe it or not, my doctor did well to convince me that was the end," said Mike, who was perhaps in his late sixties. He had been working at a construction company for over 30 years at the time of his diagnosis. The doctor affirmed that rather than mitigate, the condition was likely to get worse.

While many doctors will tell you that AFib becomes worse as you age, most are unaware of how unfriendly "worse" is. A study has confirmed that for people above sixty-five, an AFib diagnosis means that there is one out of four chances that the individual will pass away within the coming year.

Statistics have revealed a 25 percent mortality rate for people diagnosed with atrial fibrillation and that was a clarion call for Mike. It wasn't a call of despair; it was a call to make sure that every moment he has left counts. You must know that he didn't make attempts at getting healthier or better. What he wanted was to ensure that he enjoyed the time he knew he had left. So, rather than leave the doctor's office with his heart weighing down with sorrow and sadness, he chose the path of feeling positive and hopeful with great determination to improve his health and life.

He decided to quit his business. He relocated to a more serene and quiet environment. He took his medications as and when due, figuring that was the best and safer means to keep things under control. On weekends, he enjoyed the company of his grandkids and others: friends and relatives, who would show up to make him feel some sense of belonging. Unlike weekends, weekdays were boring times for him; hence, he birthed some life-changing ideas, such as going for a hike. It soon became a habit, something that, if he didn't do, he felt uneasy about. Within a couple of months, he had shed a lot of weight, although he wasn't obese. Unlike the times when he used to eat a burger and fries, dried fruits and nuts were now his favorites while hiking.

Having called it quits from his business, he had indirectly freed himself from a lot of stress. Time passed until one day, it dawned on him that it had been a long time that he hadn't had an episode of atrial fibrillation; then, he thought perhaps he had a long time to live.

Almost unintentionally, Mike was able to find hope. Several years after his first episode of atrial fibrillation, he was still in perfect health. Since it was already a habit, he never stopped hiking. He stopped taking AFib medications after that. The Mike example shows that atrial fibrillation isn't a death sentence. Life can be worth living even after the diagnosis.

Over the years, many people have lost their lives due to diseases and medical conditions related to atrial fibrillation. These people could have been assisted, if their doctors had told them to make easy and enabling changes like Mike found out on his own.

The fact remains that atrial fibrillation isn't a new phenomenon. The first known discovery of a condition, that is most probably atrial fibrillation, can be seen in a Chinese book whose origin can be dated back to as far back as 2000 years ago. "When the pulse is irregular and tremulous……..then the impulse of life fades," says Huangdi Neijing, commonly referred to as The Yellow Emperor's Classic of Medicine. It means that even before the beginning of the Qin Dynasty, which is the inception of what today is known as Imperial China, doctors seem to be associating atrial fibrillation with age and describing it as the end of all things.

As the years passed by, certain doctors found out that AFib is treatable through exercise and diet. You could say that it was so simple and clear to have been overlooked for such a long time. That's accepted. However, it doesn't look like those doctors have gotten the attention and knowledge of the medical field because historical medical books and literature on AFib lacked until the 1700s. When William Withering, an English physician, found a traditional herbal solution that he made with foxglove, the time marks the enlightenment stage. The herb was reported to be good at creating an abnormal heartbeat, more regular and complete. Later, an active chemical compound found in foxglove called digoxin was separated from it (foxglove). (You must know that most modern pharmacies still carry this chemical compound despite its gradual fall out as a contemporary treatment strategy for atrial fibrillation).

The discoveries made by Withering gave room for modern therapeutics, a thing Withering had tried to accomplish with foxglove. Thus, for centuries and years to come, researchers and medical practitioners continued searching for better, and improved pharmaceutical treatments and solutions to what many doctors seem to believe is an unavoidable condition of old age.

These opinions about AFib are perhaps overlooked by those who had no idea about what was happening inside someone's heart during an episode of atrial fibrillation. There are several theories, but it wasn't until recently (dated back to as early as the 1990s) that various research aimed to find the numerous atrial fibrillation mechanisms and the studies that include scientists inducing AFib in some organisms. Also, it contains the technology that allowed medical practitioners to look inside the human body and considerably changed perspectives and notions about the condition while having a tremendous effect on therapeutic approaches. Several years of specific knowledge about the inevitability of atrial fibrillation and taking medications to address it had metastasized by then. Hence, it is not a thing of surprise that Mike's doctor had advised him to be prepared for his burial. People diagnosed with AFib were getting similar advice at that time, and they still do today. That is very disheartening.

You might have come across the fact that about 14 percent of people diagnosed with atrial fibrillation die within a month of diagnosis. And this fact is quite scary, even because it is on well-conducted research. However, it is essential to put this number into consideration and ponder upon the context meticulously. A large number of people diagnosed with AFib are those over the age of sixty-five. Sixty-five, in this case, can be said to be hardly old, or it shouldn't be seen that way, at least. Today, many people in their mid-sixties seem to be living a healthier life than their counterparts who lived some years back. They are confident that they have more years to live without concern for any health issues.

You have maybe also learned either from personal experiences, or from a doctor, or independent research that this phenomenon of arrhythmia always comes with rapid and increasing heart rate, palpitations, chest pain, dizziness, lightheadedness, shortness of breath, or at times fainting spells. You have also probably found out that the drug and medication options for treating atrial fibrillation come with myriads of adverse side effects, more risks for other damaging conditions, and a significantly reduced quality of health and life. You may as well discover that atrial fibrillation substantially increases the chances of medical conditions such as heart failure, stroke, dementia, as well as cognitive decline. Each time an individual's heart shifts into atrial fibrillation, the blood flow rate to the brain is compromised; that is, the brain is constantly being deprived of oxygen. Due to this, the brain may eventually shrink, thereby putting the individual at risk of going through difficulties in language use, memory deficit, challenges in the way the brain process images and pictures, and problems in paying attention to details. Research has it that many of the similar biomarkers of mental injuries heightened after a concussion are as well high in AFib patients- a guide of the continuous insult of the irregular heart rhythm in the brain.

Moreover, another study showed that over 40 percent of those suffering from atrial fibrillation have traceable damage in the brain on an MRI, even if they haven't had any neurologic symptoms before. The mental changes may help explain why so many individuals have often felt quite fit and versatile to visit their doctors and medical practitioners for help. At that point, their brain can no longer work at these high rates, and their heart has an abnormal and irregular heartbeat rhythm.

Verily, the outlook of this phenomenon surely seems colorless. Hence, there is little or no wonder that researchers and experts have found out that individuals who have been diagnosed with atrial fibrillation are more likely to report a reduction in their enjoyment of recreational and leisure time. They may also complain about a decrease in the satisfaction derived while at home or work, a decline in social activities, and a significant drop in their pleasure with their sex life.

So, is there any good news for people suffering from atrial fibrillation? Of course, there is. Yes, atrial fibrillation can be the most devastating thing that has ever happened to you, yet it can also be the best. Atrial fibrillation is a warning. It is an indication that something is wrong somewhere and is even more likely to go amiss very soon. As a result of this, the health strategies offered and expounded in this piece will help you reduce and prevent the occurrence of harmful arrhythmia; they will assist you in living a happier, healthier, and longer life every day in every way.

Hence, notwithstanding several misconceptions and myths about atrial fibrillation, there is a key to living a good and healthy life with or without it. This book offers an adequate explanation of this.

As far as atrial fibrillation is concerned, your doctor may have laughed at the word "cure." You might have been told that there is no such thing as "atrial fibrillation cure." Contrarily, this is not always true.

According to different medical practitioners, the National Cancer Institute established that a cancer patient who, after being diagnosed and treated, lives for as long as five years without a recurrence could be considered to be "cured" of it. Therefore, if similar measures and standards are applied, patients diagnosed with atrial fibrillation can indeed be cured.

Without mincing words, those who achieve this goal of being cured of AFib are highly committed and recognize that it is a fight for their lives. However, it is a belief held in high esteem that as many people as are motivated can achieve this goal if they are willing and ready to comply with the treatment strategies and processes outlined in this book.

Are you feeling a bit doubtful? Perhaps a lot of doubt in your mind now. That's a positive feeling. It is no new news that the world in its whole existence doubts faith and even reality. It is much easier for people to throw concepts such as "cure" away without any regard for the harm they cause to others, especially patients who get their hopes up nonetheless, only to have them shattered on the rocks of skepticism. In the process of seeking a cure for AFib, skepticism is likely a good thing. But you must know that optimism and skepticism aren't mutually exclusive events. Science gives hope. Hence, science suggests a large room for people suffering from atrial fibrillation to feel confident and hopeful about the future, mainly when they are willing and ready to ask questions and seek answers.

What Could Cause AFib?

To many people, atrial fibrillation is a problem of the heart. But this isn't so. To better understand this, an illustration will go a long way because not everyone can relate to atrial fibrillation. For example, do you remember the last time you suffered from fever? When you have a fever, the bane of the issue is not that your body temperature had drastically risen to its peak, although that is an issue to be concerned about and a deadly one. But if your treatment, rather than been geared towards eliminating what is responsible for the fever in the first place, is directed towards reducing the high body temperature, you have just channeled your medications in the wrong direction. That is because fever is a symptom of an infection in the human body, just like atrial fibrillation is a symptom of systemic bodily disease.

When you decide to fight atrial fibrillation; you cannot just battle against the arrhythmia alone. So, if you are going to beat this thing at its game, you must know what caused it in the first instance.

Before getting acquainted with these causes, you need to know the distinction between causes and triggers. You will need to have a deep understanding of the two concepts. The long-term factors that make people vulnerable to atrial fibrillation, also referred to as substrate causes, are not often the same factors that gear a particular incident of atrial fibrillation. Using a wildfire analogy in this context may help you to understand the differences better. A spark can trigger a single blaze, but the chances of having a lot of fires at a time are greatly influenced by factors including an infestation of insects, drought, as well as underbrush growth. Hence, the substrate causes and not just the triggers of atrial fibrillation must be carefully examined.

When doctors tell their patients about some substrate causes of AFib, they are always surprised. Some even show anger in the process.

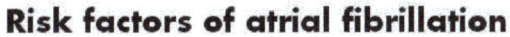

Risk factors of atrial fibrillation

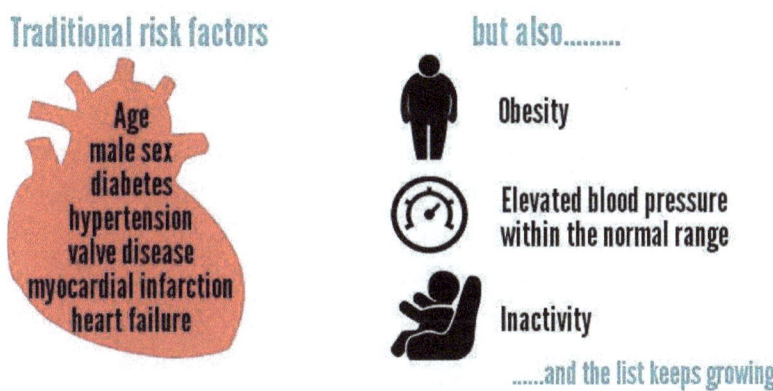

"I know I can't hide it, right? I've made a lot of bad decisions as regards my health and choice of food," said a working-class woman named Debbie as she remembered her first visit to a doctor during her atrial fibrillation diagnosis.

"But it looked like my doctor was committed to forcing me to tell him about those things. Although I felt guilty, yet all I desired was getting whatever drugs I needed, or take whatever steps I needed to take, leaving myself little time to think about the horrible things I may have done to my family or even to myself".

It is unlikely to know if Debbie's doctor had approached her with the accurate and decisively elusive combination of compassion and confidence that is often referred to as the "bedside manners" of a physician. However, what can be deduced is that if your focus lies on fighting atrial fibrillation, rather than treating and waiting for it to deteriorate as time passes by, you need to understand the root factors that cause the disease.

Despite the many available technologies and sciences, many doctors still tell people diagnosed with AFib that nothing can be done about it and that there is little they can do now but worsen the situation. So, they end up prescribing some drugs or call up several steps, and that's the end of it. However, rather than curing the condition with pharmaceutical medications or treating only the most apparent symptoms, the best course of action is to look out for the specific and unique underlying causes in order to keep it from resurfacing. Often, that cause is a combination of different reasons and may not be the same with every individual. No two persons can end up having atrial fibrillation for the exact same reasons.

Debbie now understands this better.

"Now that I have more knowledge about atrial fibrillation, I see my initial visit to my physician differently," said Debbie. "If I had just used whatever drugs he gave me or follow the list of steps he related and didn't pay close attention to the root factors that led me to have atrial fibrillation in the first instance, I wouldn't have experienced any change. Instead, I might have felt better and healthier for some time, and then things likely might have taken the wrong bend afterwards".

Everyone, no one is exempted here, has made wrong decisions about their health and choice of food at one time or another. Although we have easy access to research papers and training on atrial fibrillation, the list does not exclude doctors who still develop the condition. Therefore, it is not surprising at all to meet a physician, in fact, a cardiologist, who has had to fight this condition.

With that in mind, kindly understand that the exercise that follows in the later paragraphs of this section will be asked to assess the various causes of your atrial fibrillation, and it isn't a guilt attempt. Instead, it is an integral part of building a treatment plan that is suitable for you.

So, why did you have AFib? Many substrate causes could be responsible for this, some of which you can and cannot control. Some of the reasons why you have atrial fibrillation include the following:

You Inherited the Gene from Your Parents

More often than not, many people inherit the wrong genetic predisposition that makes them vulnerable to atrial fibrillation. In addition, research has shown that up to a third of AFib victims without another known cause have a familial history of the disease.

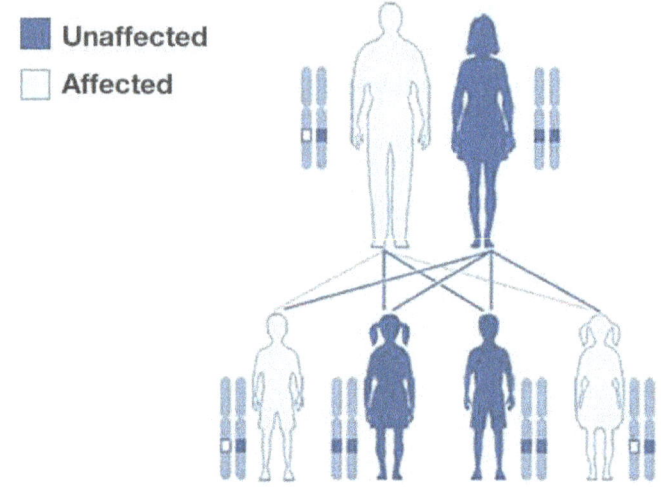

This association is not self-oriented. Instead, it relates to a gene called KCNQ1. This gene acts as a form of instruction paper for building and developing vital components of the heart muscle cells responsible for transporting potassium ions. Numerically, not less than fifteen various "potassium channel" mutations have been attributed to atrial fibrillation.

Another type of gene on which experts and researchers are incredibly focused is the SCNA5, which affects the ability of the body to transport sodium ions. Numerically, not less than seven "sodium channel" mutations have been attributed to atrial fibrillation.

Sodium and potassium ions are atoms that electric transport charges and, for that reason, are vital to the signaling system that informs parts of the heart to reduce in rhythm. But, contrary to this, several non-ion-channel mutations have been said to be associated with atrial fibrillation. These include mutations in a gene called LMNA that is related to disorders of the heart, a protein-coding gene known as NUP155, a gene referred to as NPPA that encodes a vital hormone secreted in the heart, and a group of genes called GATA6, GATA5, and GATA6 that are essential for the development of new heart cells and tissues.

It doesn't end there. Many other genes have been attributed to atrial fibrillation, and more than a hundred of them. If the list continued, it would be counterproductive because it would very soon be old and outdated. An emerging study is showing other "possible genes" that may be associated with atrial fibrillation. However, for now, no test or scan can reveal all the potential and known "Atrial Fibrillation Genes." While some products, such as the over-the-counter DNA tests, will scan for some, you are just scratching the surface with them.

What is imperative for you to consider is that while it can be safer to know if you have inherited genetic susceptibility to atrial fibrillation, you can do nothing about the genes you have.

On the other hand, it is also necessary for you to know that research carried out over the past few years in epigenetics has finally demonstrated that every individual has the power to impact "suppressed" and "expressed" genes based on their daily health decisions and choices. Indeed, health outcomes/results amongst people who have inherited these genes vary significantly depending on factors that go far beyond the inheritance.

You Are Suffering From another Heart Problem

If you were to look at all the people suffering from atrial fibrillation across the globe, you would find out that more than half of them have been diagnosed with a different cardiovascular infection. Of all these infections, the three top culprits include coronary artery infection, cardiac valve problem, and heart failure.

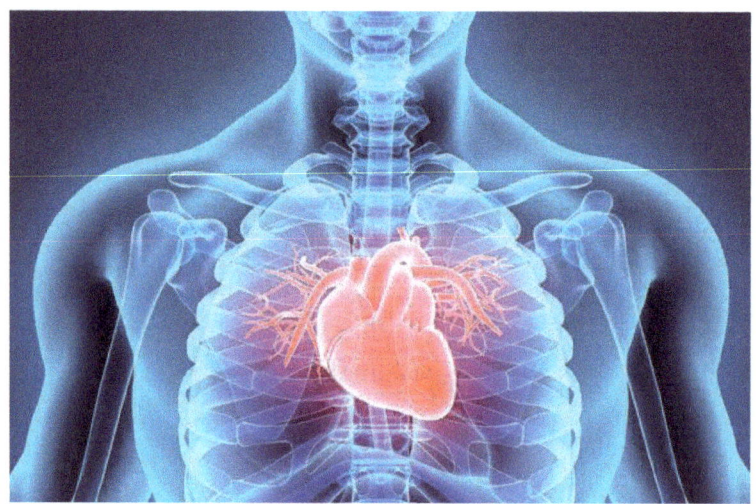

Kelvin had no idea what was wrong with him. He decided to go for a medical check-up. Not only did he find out that he had atrial fibrillation that had been going on for several months, but he was also having health issues like heart failure as well as coronary artery disease. Some years back, Kelvin had been stented for a blockage of the artery. But very recently, he developed rapid atrial fibrillation, which caused his heart to be beating at the rate of 140 beats per minute. Of course, for individuals who are often engaged in strenuous exercises, this heartbeat rate can still be said to be expected. But that wasn't the only problem he was confronting.

"I needed not to be told that things were beginning to get awkward," Kelvin said. "They all appear in their numbers one after the other; shortness of breath, chest pains, palpitations and several others that I can't seem to be able to mention. I was losing it rapidly".

Kelvin, unfortunately, was suffering from a lot of heart problems at the same time. Thus, there was a need for him to put an end to his long-term atrial fibrillation medications. Failure to do this would subject him to dangerous side effects, increasing the risk of adverse outcomes associated with other heart issues.

There wasn't anything he could do at the time to curtail the damage his other heart problems were inflicting on his heart. So, how did he survive it? You're surely eager to know how he sailed through it and came out healthy, aren't you? His unwavering commitment to the strategies provided and expounded in this book aided his recovery from AFib and other heart problems.

The Age Factor

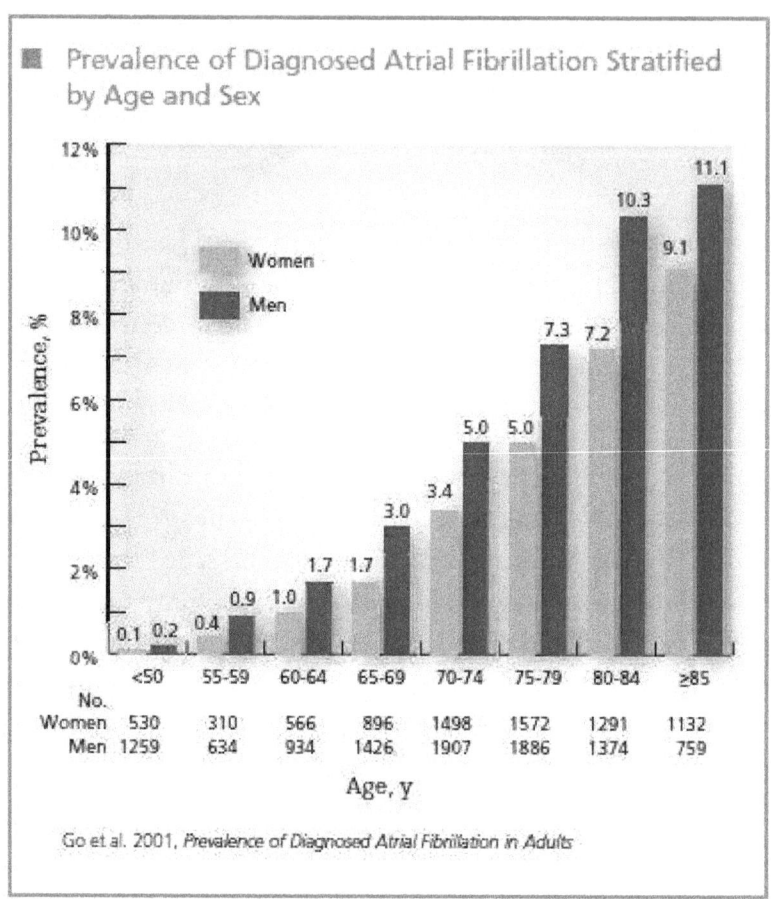

Prevalence of Diagnosed Atrial Fibrillation Stratified by Age and Sex

	<50	55-59	60-64	65-69	70-74	75-79	80-84	≥85
No. Women	530	310	566	896	1498	1572	1291	1132
Men	1259	634	934	1426	1907	1886	1374	759

Go et al. 2001, *Prevalence of Diagnosed Atrial Fibrillation in Adults*

Living a healthy life has become a habit for some people. They are so meticulous about their health and energy that they make choices to stay healthy. Their selection of food, drink, snacks, as well as the drugs they use is well pondered upon.

Such was the life of Barbara. She had stayed healthy her whole life. She had stayed off fast, processed, and fried foods and solely depended on a plant-based diet. She avoided the consumption of sugar and any other sugary substance. As a result, she did not tend to be obese or overweight. She took part in aerobics now and then in the gym and turned yoga class into an everyday thing. Whenever her stress levels began to increase rapidly, she would start her deep-breathing exercises to reduce the effects. As a result, she always had enough sleep at night. More interestingly, she willingly consented to work as a crosswalk guard somewhere around where her house was situated.

Upon her doctor telling her that she had an irregularity in the rate of heartbeats (arrhythmia), she was more than irritated since none of her family members had ever suffered from atrial fibrillation. So, what could have been wrong?

The thing is, Barbara wasn't on the good side of age again. She was in her mid-nineties. Thus, doing all the activities and engaging in various exercises and being careful enough not to eat processed or fast foods, do not eliminate the chances of having atrial fibrillation. Age is one factor that increases the risks of having AFib. The older you are, the more susceptible you are to having it. Just as your skin would get wrinkled as you age, simply living your life will place some wear and tear on the cells and tissues of your heart over time.

There is also the concept of premature ageing. But, of course, there is a vast difference between being ninety-five and being fifty or sixty. Therefore, there is a type of atrial fibrillation that arises naturally due to old age and that which comes up because of premature ageing. And since you have no right over the number of candles on your birthday cake (concerning chronological age), there are a lot of things you can choose to do to put your biological ageing process under control.

What are the things you need to do to slow down or turn back your biological age? Knowing what to do will reduce your vulnerability to AFib. The procedures in this piece will not only help you to fight against atrial fibrillation, but they will also help you to know what steps to take to slow down your biological age.

High Blood Pressure

You know what this is, don't you? You know what this is likely to cause if you do not manage or have it controlled? One of the dangers of having high blood pressure, and probably the most evident, is hypertension. You are said to have had hypertension when the force of your blood against the walls of one's arteries is high to the extent that it puts you at risk of severe health problems. Taking a critical look at the heart, you will observe that the heart is works tirelessly to pump blood via very restrictive arteries with each heartbeat. Combining this strain and stress can lead to the enlargement and unhealthy thickness of the heart muscles. The result of this is a disruption of electrical pathways which ultimately results in atrial fibrillation. In fact, of all the factors that have been said to be responsible for causing atrial fibrillation, there is none as potent as hypertension.

You're still not getting the equation. OK, here it is. High blood pressure is a significant cause of hypertension which, according to research, is the most frequently encountered condition in people suffering from atrial fibrillation. Research has also shown that high blood pressure and hypertension nearly doubles the chances of having AFib. Studies have also shown that about 90 percent of the United States inhabitants are vulnerable to hypertension by the age of fifty-five. Thus, there is little or no wonder about why atrial fibrillation is so common.

This situation has not always been the style of things. For example, just about 4 percent of the centenarians residing in the famed "Longevity Village" of Bapan, a place in the Southern part of China, were known to be victims of high blood pressure. There is also a similar study that borders around hunter-gatherers who lived in the rainforest of the Amazon. These hunter-gatherers showed a natural and consistent blood pressure of about 110/70 which does not rise except age. It seems from many studies and research that the genes in the human body are created to keep blood pressure in the 110/70 natural range without drugs and in as much as you don't make things worse with your carefree contemporary lifestyle.

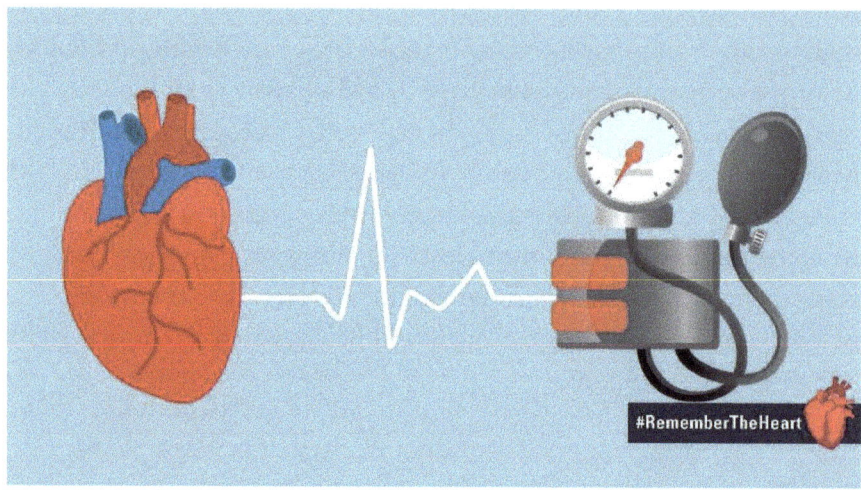

How these groups of people were able to achieve this is very clear and simple. They chose plant-based diets over fast and processed foods and sugar. That's not all. They watched their weight as they grew, made physical exercise a daily routine, cultivated the act of having sound and sufficient sleep, and tried, by all means possible, to reduce their stress levels. All these things reduced their chances of having hypertension.

Living such a life in this modern time can be pretty challenging due to humans' different innovations and inventions to make life easy and stress-free.

However, one can say that it is not feasible. There are myriads of lessons from the lifestyle these people chose for themselves, and if you are not limited by imagination, you can heal by applying some of these lessons to your own life.

Drug/Medication Effects

You should meet Fagin. Fagin was in his late forties. He had a well-paying job and a son who made him happy now and then. He loved music and, for that reason, got engaged with his community singers' group. No day passed by without him going out for exercise. From a distance, you could see that he was fit. His fitness wasn't just a result of his daily routine; it was also a result of the many track and field events he did. He took part in running activities in his community. The idea of processed or fast food was unfriendly to him. He preferred plant-based foods. He ensured he had enough sleep each night to avoid any complications. Fagin was quite acquainted with atrial fibrillation. A friend of his, to whom he was very close, had an episode of AFib, and it was during this incidence that he got to know the basic things about the medical condition.

"It caught me unaware like I wasn't even sure that was me," he said, "because when this thing happened to my friend, I had learned that staying healthy was an effective way to prevent it, even as far as those who got it from their parents are concerned. Just stay healthy, and that was all. But just in a split of a second, I was sitting in my parlor when suddenly my heartbeat started going up, up, and up. I was shocked this was happening to me. I knew what it was because it had happened to my friend; it didn't just make sense to me". I listened to him intently as he spoke about his experience.

Although it didn't make any sense to Fagin at first, he later realized that there was a lot of sense in it. That's because since he had been diagnosed to be hypertensive in his middle thirties, he had resorted to taking hydrochlorothiazide, commonly referred to as HCTZ. HCTZ is a popular diuretic that physicians always prescribe to assist their patients in controlling the risk of high blood pressure.

But, unfortunately, further diagnosis showed that Fagin's body had suffered significant depletion of minerals like magnesium and potassium due to HCTZ.

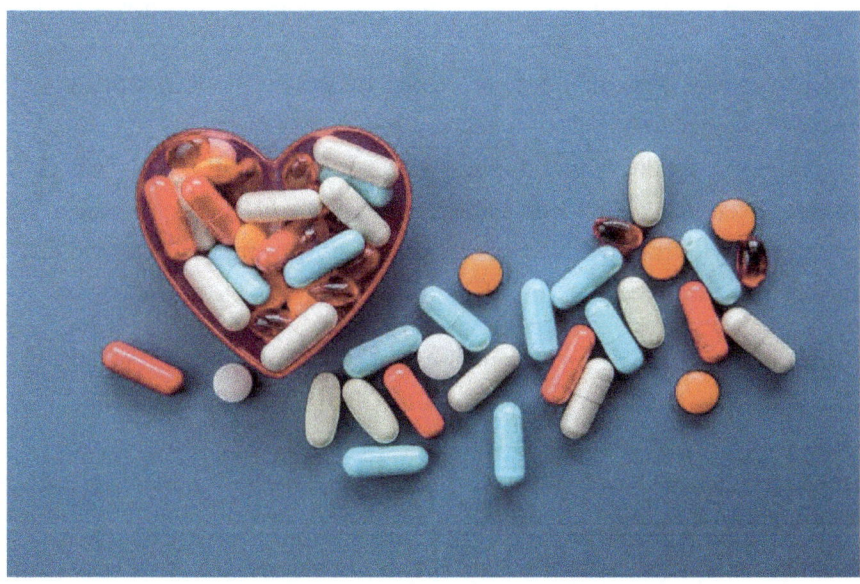

The question now is what was responsible for Fagin's atrial fibrillation? Was it his medications, high blood pressure, hypertension, or something else they couldn't diagnose? While high blood pressure is a significant factor that one may liken to his condition, it is also possible that the hydrochlorothiazide had caused a trigger due to the low level of magnesium and potassium. In my experience, most cases of AFib induced by medications are as a result of taking one or more harmful drugs in addition to other atrial fibrillation risk factors. However, because Fagin was fit and hardly ate foods that could heighten his risk of having AFib, it was probably surfacing in the arrhythmias he was having.

"It was funny to me anyway," he recounted. "I wasn't expecting it to happen to me. One of the major reasons I took to doing exercises every day and being watchful of what I consumed was my experience with hypertension. Apart from the little aspirin I was taking to deal with the headache, this was the only medication I was taking, and I think it increased my chances of having AFib".

It wasn't indispensable for Fagin to be taking hydrochlorothiazide anymore because his blood pressure had long fallen to a considerably healthy level. Hence, rather than the HCTZ, it was the regular exercise, good sleep habits, low body weight, diet, and no-stress lifestyle that he cultivated had helped him maintain stable blood pressure levels.

Diuretics of hydrochlorothiazide such as HTCZ are not the only drugs that are associated with atrial fibrillation. Medications like NSAIDs (Nonsteroidal anti-inflammatory drugs) can also cause AFib. Medicines that belong to this category include naproxen and ibuprofen that are always taken to treat pains. These drugs (nonsteroidal anti-inflammatory drugs) are potential risks for having AFib as they extensively make patients susceptible to kidney and heart failure. In addition, life-threatening medical conditions like gastro-intestinal bleeding can also be caused by NSAIDs, particularly for people on blood thinners.

If you are used to taking Proton-pump inhibitors, you might be increasing your chances of having irregular heartbeats. This is because these medications limit stomach acid and induce arrhythmia by hindering magnesium absorption or altering an individual's gut microbiome. These medications include pantoprazole, lansoprazole, and omeprazole. They are usually sold under the brand tags Protonix, Prevacid, and Prilosec, respectively.

Steroids such as methylprednisolone and prednisone are also potential causes of AFib. They increase blood pressure rapidly and push blood glucose levels very high via weight gain and retention.

That list hasn't ended. As far back as the early 2000s, a group of researchers led by Bruno Stricker, an epidemiologist, started to conduct studies to explore and discover drugs that could be associated with AFib. They found out that cardiac stimulant drugs had been linked with atrial fibrillation. Even counter-placed decongestants like pseudoephedrine, which is offered for sale as Sudafed, and medications for hyperactivity/attention-deficit disorder can cause an attack of AFib to be triggered.

Also, some classic medications used for treating irregular heart rhythms (calcium and digoxin channel blockers like diltiazem and verapamil) can cause atrial fibrillation. Stricker's team also noted that many emphysema and asthma drugs had been associated with AFib. Stimulant inhalers such as albuterol and theophylline derived from xanthine are included in this list.

Central nervous system medications include antidepressants such as fluoxetine (commonly referred to as Prozac); anti-migraine drugs such as sumatriptan (much more popularly called by the name Imitrex); and dopamine agonists (apomorphine), which is used for treating Parkinson's disease. These examples and Anticholinergics, which are occasionally used instead of antipsychotics to treat Parkinson's disease, can trigger AFib. Worse still, doctors usually prescribed drugs such as beta-blockers to treat atrial fibrillation can be associated with AFib episodes. It is primarily due to weight gain, especially in women.

Dated to 2004, Stricker and his group of researchers discovered case studies and reports that connect AFib to more than fifty-eight prescription medications. Every year after then, several drugs associated with atrial fibrillation have been included in the list.

For instance, a few years after reports that some anti-osteoporosis drugs such as Fosamax could cause a trigger of AFib, hundreds of thousands of women grew concerns about them as a result of the report. Luckily, during a study of not less than 40,000 people, it was discovered that bisphosphonates (a type of medication) have no association with atrial fibrillation. Hence, it can be said that every drug ought to be tested and evaluated to determine if at all it can trigger AFib.

Don't be caught off guard, for the fact that a drug has been linked to being responsible for atrial fibrillation doesn't mean that you shouldn't take it. If your doctor prescribed it, you could go-ahead to use it. After all, all types of medications have potential side effects. The safest way to make decisions about prescribed drugs is to ask questions. If you would like to know how some of the drugs impact you; you should ask your physician that question. No condition should tempt you to use drugs that have been prescribed to you without the guidance and knowledge of your doctor. Suppose you have been diagnosed with atrial fibrillation, or perhaps you think you might be susceptible to it. In that case, you should do well to inform your physician about every type of drug that you are taking, both occasional counter-placed and common medications.

Life has been made easy. Just a simple internet search for the concept "AFib" and the name of the medication you are taking can relate to you if there's any association between the drug and AFib. Interestingly, both the famous and less popular potential side effects of all medicines are made available from several reputable sources such as the US Foods and Drug Administration. It means that you don't necessarily need to book an appointment with your doctor to have this information at your disposal. But it is indispensable to see your doctor in some cases.

Many people make a mistake while telling their doctors about the drugs they are taking when they leave the supplements out. They often see no reason to tell their doctors about them, perhaps because they think these supplements are less critical. Many don't even see vitamins and other supplements as drugs. However, like any therapy type, one should only take the proper doses of these supplements for the right purpose and time. Research has found out that individuals who take vitamin D, for instance, are two and a half times more vulnerable to having an AFib attack.

Concerning atrial fibrillation, the mechanism of action of one medication varies from the other. Therefore, let's take a cursory look at some of these drugs and their means of activities.

- **Stimulants:** irrespective of their types, they are responsible for increasing blood pressure levels and the release of adrenaline.
- **Anti-arrhythmics**: some of these medications trigger changes in electrical conduction in the heart.
- **Diuretics:** any of these drugs can cause dehydration and depletion of electrolytes.
- **Nonsteroidal Inflammatory Drugs (NSAIDs)** such as naproxen and ibuprofen can increase blood pressure levels. They also cause fluid retention.
- **Amiodarone:** This is a type of drug that causes thyroid hormones to be released. Too much thyroid hormone can be a stimulant.
- **Nicotine:** This medication acts as a stimulant that causes inflammation from vaping and cardiac toxicity.
- **Steroids:** They are also responsible for the increase in blood pressure and retention of body fluid.
- **Proton-pump inhibitors** such as Protonix, Prevacid, and Prilosec: Hinder magnesium in the gut.

- **Marijuana:** This has myriads of effects. First, it leads to changes in the autonomic nervous system. Second, it is also responsible for the inadequate flow of blood to the heart.
- **Alcohol:** Some of the mechanisms of action associated with alcohol are sleep disorder, weight gain, cardiac toxicity, and an increase in the levels of blood pressure.

You are eating too much-processed food and sugar.

Are you looking for good medicine? Then food is one. A diet that honors what is required by the body to survive might be the safest way to prevent AFib, or better still, fight against it once its rear it appears. But, unfortunately, the exact opposite is what you are likely to get if you choose a terrible diet. There isn't anything that is as bad and risky as feeding on processed foods and sugar as far as atrial fibrillation is concerned, to be candid.

You should do away with foods containing high amounts of sugar like candies, pastries, confections, and sodas. The hidden fact many people are not used to is their failure to recognize that many of the foods they think are healthy are often packed with a lot of sugar. When the word "sugar" is mentioned, it goes beyond the tiny brown or white granules added to morning coffee or used for baking, although it can also include this. This ordinary sugar is what is known as sucrose. Apart from this, there are about five other types of sugar. They is fructose, glucose, maltose, lactose, and galactose. Due to this, even cautious "label readers" may not be aware that the foods they are buying and consuming have added sugar concealed in the supposedly healthy ingredients such as honey, agave, juice, rice syrup, nectar, and barley malt. However, irrespective of the name they bear, they have similar adverse effects on the body. A sudden compression of sugar courses via the blood can result in instability of blood levels which can cause cardiac scarring, which, when given a little time or more, can deteriorate into AFib.

Another huge supplier of carbs in many individual foods is refined cereals like white rice and white flour, which have lost their natural nutritional value and fibers. The equation is quite simple to grasp.

The more you process a grain, the faster it digests to form sugar. Another consequence that you are likely to suffer is feeling hungry shortly after eating these food substances.

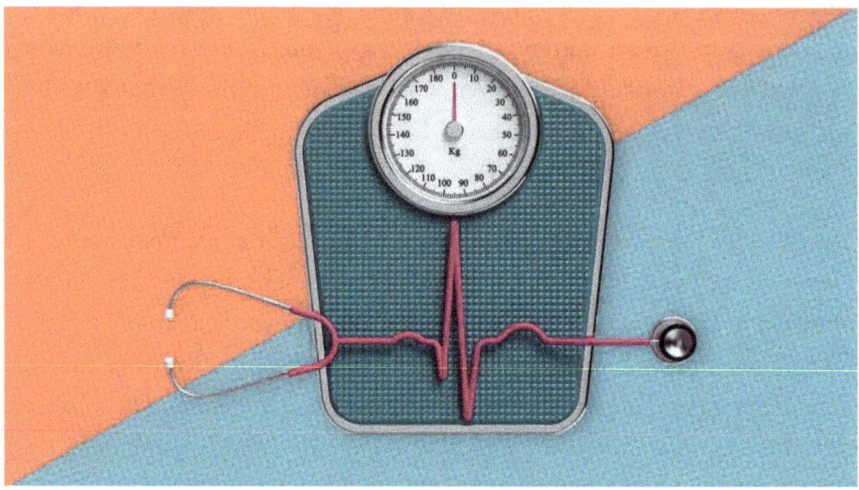

You won't feel full even after taking a whole lot of these foods. More painfully, not even a whole wheat bread can do you better. When compared to Snickers bar, a single slice of wheat bread can increase your blood glucose drastically.

All these notions put together do not mean that you should avoid taking sugar. That is not the point. However, specific experts believe that in trying to reduce the amount of sugar in your body, a deficient diet may be very detrimental and heighten your risks of atrial fibrillation. Thus, the bone of contention here is that you must ensure that, to the most outstanding level possible, the carbohydrates you are eating are Complex carbs, like vegetables and fruits.

At this point, you should be able to carry out a realistic assessment of your eating habits and link them to processed foods and sugar. For example, suppose you are not disciplined enough to avoid consuming processed foods and foods with high amounts of sugar and carbohydrates to foods decorated with complex carbohydrates (fruits and vegetables). In that case, you might be exposing yourself to episodes of atrial fibrillation.

You are getting little or No Exercise.

Benefits of Exercise Training in AF

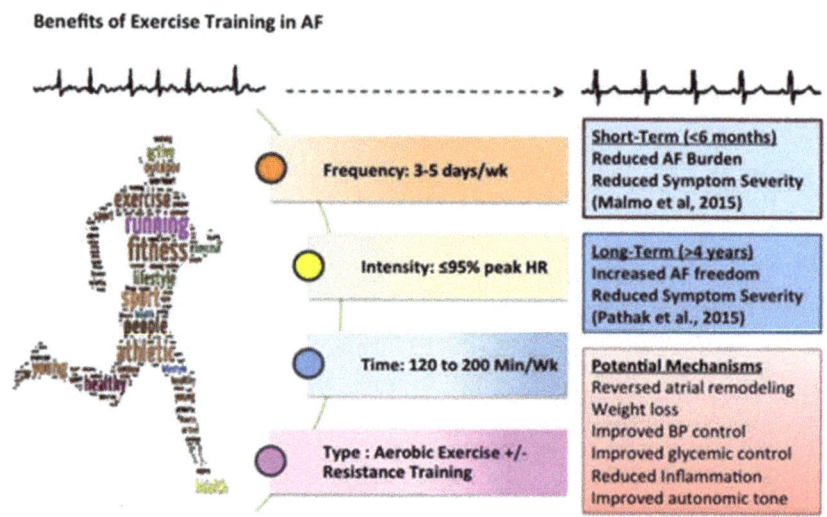

● Frequency: 3-5 days/wk		**Short-Term (<6 months)** Reduced AF Burden Reduced Symptom Severity (Malmo et al, 2015)
● Intensity: ≤95% peak HR		**Long-Term (>4 years)** Increased AF freedom Reduced Symptom Severity (Pathak et al., 2015)
● Time: 120 to 200 Min/Wk		**Potential Mechanisms** Reversed atrial remodeling Weight loss Improved BP control Improved glycemic control Reduced Inflammation Improved autonomic tone
● Type : Aerobic Exercise +/- Resistance Training		

The first time Fagin related to me that he was a runner, all I wanted to know was the running he did.

"So which one did you specialize in, relay, a hundred meters, marathon, or other little stuff?" I asked him.

"Well, when I was much younger, say in my mid-teens to my mid-twenties, I took part in many long-distance races, even marathon," Fagin said. "Just a few years ago, I took part in my first triathlon, and to be candid; it wasn't like I had much interest in these events, I did them for the sake of my health, so, for now, I prefer short distance races to the long ones. But if you think I need more of that to stay healthy, I have no other option than to-------"

"Not at all. You don't need to," I interrupted. "My concern isn't that you aren't running as much as you should do; rather, you're having an attack of atrial fibrillation could have been as a result of too much running," I concluded.

Over the years, it has been discovered that people who engage in ultra-endurance and long-distance activities such as cross-country skiing, biking, and running have high risks of suffering from at least one attack of atrial fibrillation in their lifetime. Fagin was appalled, and so was everyone who for the first time knew that persons who engage in a competitive cycle, or run marathons, or do triathlons are five times more susceptible to have AFib. The significant part is that studies have not shown that athletes who take part in highly strenuous activities such as weightlifting, wrestling, and boxing have higher chances of developing arrhythmias. However, there is something peculiar about endurance activities that heighten the risk of having AFib. (One activity that is exempted from this list is football. Even among former NFL players, the chances of having atrial fibrillation are six times higher. However, this may be due to using performance-enhancing drugs or the weight of some players to perform at professional levels).

Moreover, it is vital to note that while actively participating in endurance activities may increase your risk of having atrial fibrillation, participating in them does not mean developing AFib. It is interesting also to know that recreational engagement in endurance activities, even if it is a triathlon or marathon, doesn't increase the risk. Frequent and regular exercise has nothing to do with this; the body needs to stay healthy. To make things more transparent, for every thousand patients diagnosed with atrial fibrillation, perhaps just one of them has suffered AFib due to over-exercising. The most devastating problem is that many patients do not have sufficient exercise.

There are far more risks from not exercising at all than from having too much exercise. For example, people who exhibit sedentary habits are more vulnerable to atrial fibrillation, not to talk of many other health complications.

You Are Not Getting Enough Sleep

Whenever there are concerns to get healthier, and irrespective of why you have chosen to do that, you more than often start with exercise and diet, thus, neglecting the sleep factor. Although diet and exercise are two essential factors, people tend to overlook the third factor: sufficient sleep, which without it, you won't notice any significant improvement.

A large number of the population does not get sufficient sleep. And as a global village, it would appear that instead of improving in this regard, things are becoming worse, even as science and technology, which ought to offer solutions to most of our problems, have taken their toll on our everyday life. The WHO (World Health Organization) has raised concerns that the phenomenon of inadequate sleep will become a global epidemic sooner than expected. For instance, in the United States, about 70 percent of the seniors were reported to have an insufficient sleep at least twice a month, and an average of 12 percent was said to have inadequate sleep every night.

Between 2004 and 2012 (eight years), the period witnessed a significant level of people who were having less than 6 hours of sleep.

Another shock was released when a demographic sociologist and his team looked into the topic. Yes, the period between 2004 and 2012 saw a great level out, but from 2013 to 2017, there was a significant shift. A lot of people were reported to be having insufficient sleep.

So, what changed? Among the most commonly responsible factors are the accessories we regularly carry about in our purses and pockets and other devices. Closely colliding with the dropping rate of sufficient sleep was the increase in smartphones, which increasing from 35 percent as of 2011 to 78 percent by 2016. "A large number of Americans now spend several hours looking at screens," Connor and his team reported, "and as a result of the mobile nature of these accessories, technology has gradually found its way into the bedroom."

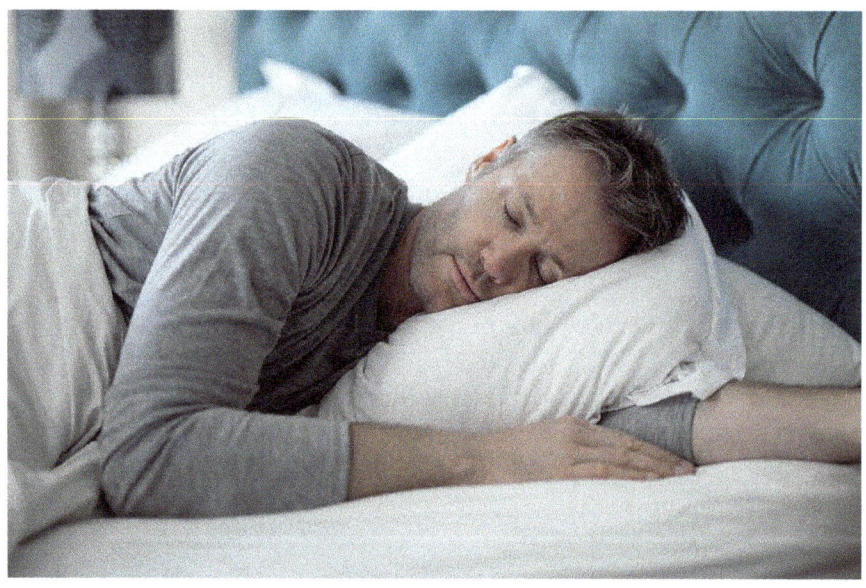

It isn't a phenomenon peculiar to the United States. It's the same across the globe. Taking a closer look at world facts, more than six billion people globally now have mobile accessories, and more than half of these accessories are smartphones. Topping the table of countries using these bright screens is North Korea, where relatively 95 percent of adults have a mobile phone and where, maybe coincidentally, adults have almost forty minutes less sleep every night. That is on average in comparison with people living in other parts of the world. Since these devices are potential causes of insufficient sleep, and as they have become so equipped to fathom the health complications that come with inadequate sleep, it shouldn't be a surprise to know that cases of atrial fibrillation are skyrocketing in North Korea.

The effects of inadequate sleep on atrial fibrillation have been well-taken note of. Even minimal interruptions of sleep duration and quality can heighten the risk of AFib by 47 percent. People who suffer from insomnia have been said to be 36 percent more susceptible to having atrial fibrillation. People who do not sleep deeply: the kind of sleep that guarantees stable health, are 18 percent more at risk of suffering AFib.

People battling with a sleep disorder are 200 to 400 percent more vulnerable to having atrial fibrillation than people without a sleep disorder. The complex part of this is that once atrial fibrillation develops, poor sleep quality can be heightened by three to four times the average rate due to the presence of an irregular rhythm.

Apart from the devastating experience of not feeling well-rested, lack of sufficient sleep can also result in excess adrenaline and cortisol release. What happens with cortisol is that it helps you retain water, thereby losing potassium and increasing your blood pressure and blood sugar levels. Adrenaline, similar to what happens with cortisol, forces the heart to work much harder by increasing blood pressure. In addition, intravenous adrenaline is often used to cause a trigger of an episode of atrial fibrillation to determine the affected spot in a patient's heart.

As things would turn out, later on, I discovered that one of the underlying factors responsible for Debbie's diagnosis was sleep.

"To me, having a deep sleep, let's say for 8 hours each night, was similar to laziness", she said. "I mean, I had a lot to do at the time. I wanted to be a good and responsive mother to my two kids, to my students at college; I made sure I led by example by making sure that I was punctual for school every day. I attended church activities; I was there too to contribute my part. My favourite sport was tennis, and I also made time for that. I was proud of my lifestyle". So, what did she later find out? She found out that her consistent lack of sleep was responsible for her development of AFib. She was in her late forties at this period.

"Once my heart began to beat irregularly, I knew the problem had started. It was shocking to me to be sincere", she recounted. "The effects were many. I had to quit tennis; being a good and punctual teacher became complicated to do. To an extent, being a good mom wasn't hard for me; it all feels normal when my kids are around me. The big fear was making myself more susceptible to heart attack, stroke, and all kinds of other medical complications that could have hindered my healthy life and probably cut my life short".

Sleep wasn't just a contributive factor to Debbie's development of atrial fibrillation; it was also necessary for her full recovery. Once you can get enough sleep, and as they say, "better sleep," you will "win in the end."

You Are Consuming Too Much Alcohol and Energy Drinks.

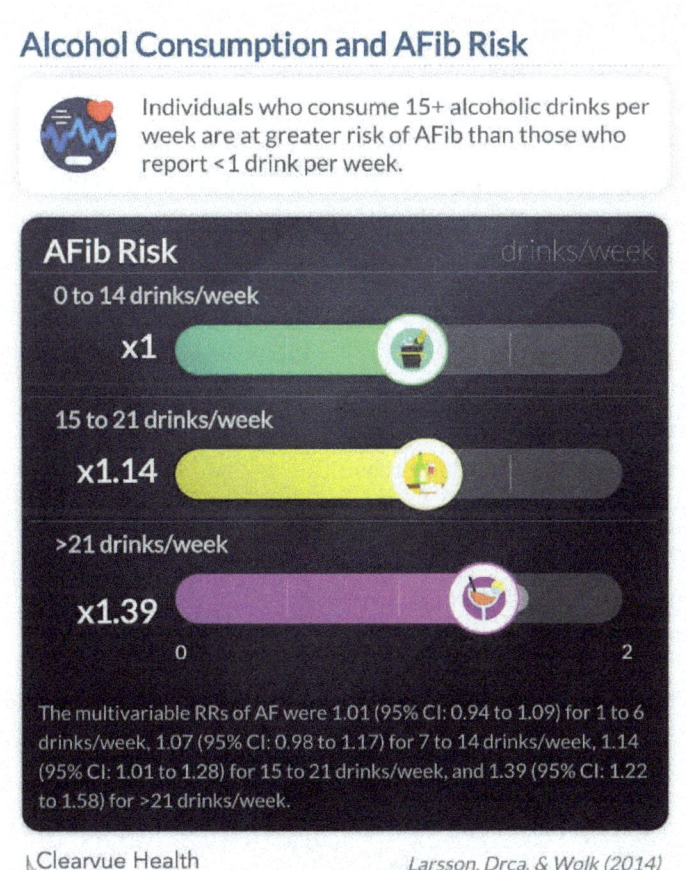

Alcohol Consumption and AFib Risk

Individuals who consume 15+ alcoholic drinks per week are at greater risk of AFib than those who report <1 drink per week.

AFib Risk drinks/week

0 to 14 drinks/week
x1

15 to 21 drinks/week
x1.14

>21 drinks/week
x1.39

0   2

The multivariable RRs of AF were 1.01 (95% CI: 0.94 to 1.09) for 1 to 6 drinks/week, 1.07 (95% CI: 0.98 to 1.17) for 7 to 14 drinks/week, 1.14 (95% CI: 1.01 to 1.28) for 15 to 21 drinks/week, and 1.39 (95% CI: 1.22 to 1.58) for >21 drinks/week.

Clearvue Health   *Larsson, Drca, & Wolk (2014)*

If you are perhaps looking for a busy woman, you should meet Gina. She was a mother of three kids who were still in elementary school. She took the job of a part-time basketball coach to complement her work as a financial secretary in the travel industry.

She also acted as president of the parent-teacher forum at her kid's school. She was pretty engaged. Being up and active in all these areas meant she would have some early mornings and late nights.

She soon found a solution to her problems of weakness and fatigue. Each time she felt stressed, she would resort to taking energy drinks, and before she could realize it, these drinks began to take their toll on her.

For some categories of people suffering from atrial fibrillation, caffeine isn't an issue. Reports have shown that the caffeine contained in tea, coffee, and chocolate does not trigger atrial fibrillation in most people. Even though sugar-enriched soda pop has been associated with diabetes, weight gain, and hypertension (even artificially sugar-enriched soda pop can be an issue), these drinks have little or no connection with AFib. However, a combination or mixture of caffeine with other stimulants like those used in energy drinks may increase the risk of AFib. Also, if your caffeine intake is what keeps you awake at night, you should know that it is detrimental to not just your sleep but also to your general wellbeing. It could also aggravate your risk of suffering atrial fibrillation.

Another factor that made things complicated in Gina's case was genetics. She had a variant CYPIA2 gene that indicates the rate at which caffeine is metabolized in her body. The effect of this was that after a long and tiring day, she usually couldn't sleep. Her body could metabolize all those rising methylxanthine chemicals quickly.

As time passed by, she had cases of heart palpitations. These heart palpitations made her stay awake every night. Her lack of sleep complicated the whole thing. She had no other option than to visit her doctor to determine what the problem was. She was later diagnosed with intermittent atrial fibrillation; an unstable heart condition medically referred to as paroxysmal atrial fibrillation. She attempted to put up with it for some time but couldn't as her condition worsened.

Consequently, even after they told her that her high consumption of energy drinks was responsible for her atrial fibrillation attack, Gina still couldn't quit the habit. It was already an everyday habit. The truth is, there are a lot of people like Gina. According to research conducted by the John Hopkins University School of Medicine, more than half of the United States inhabitants have an unquenchable taste for caffeine or have not been able to reduce their intake of caffeine. Similarly, the researchers discovered that one in every eight Americans continue to take caffeine even after knowing that the substance was doing a lot of harm to their health, including worsening insomnia, stoking anxiety, and aggravating hypertension. Well, this is just as far as caffeine is concerned. In several energy drinks, caffeine is often mixed with other ingredients like guarana, taurine, ginkgo Biloba, glucuronolactone, ginseng, and many more.

However, in Gina's case, the good news was that she didn't drink alcohol. Taking alcohol could have increased her risk of developing atrial fibrillation extensively, even if the quantity consumed was as little as drinking one unit per day. Alcohol is responsible for the formation of scar tissue in the heart. It can as well damage the electrical pathways leading to the core.

It may interest you to know that alcohol consumption does not only increase your chances of having atrial fibrillation; it also exposes you to developing life-threatening medical conditions such as cancer. And while some researchers have suggested that a bit of alcohol could be beneficial to your body, those benefits are surpassed by the high risk of developing other health-related complications. According to the 2018 study conducted by "The Lancet," the impeccable British medical journal had no controversial issues. "The conclusions of the study are clear and transparent enough," the authors scripted. In addition to this conclusion was a guideline written by the chief medical officer of the United Kingdom, which read "no safe level of the consumption of alcohol."

There is a clear difference in health outcomes between individuals who consume the once-in-a-while alcohol beverage and those who consume it in large quantity.

However, if you aim to know why you may be vulnerable to developing AFib, either for present or future risks, this is clear enough: energy drinks are detrimental to your health. Also, alcohol, irrespective of how small the quantity, can heighten your risk.

You Either Smoke or Live in a Polluted Environment

Researchers and experts have discovered gaseous pollutants usually found in toxic air to become more adverse with every passing hour. They can increase the vulnerability for deadly diseases and infections. At the zenith of these fatal diseases is atrial fibrillation. There is a massive connection between AFib and these gaseous pollutants.

Can polluted air cause individual atrial fibrillation? The answer to this question was the bone of contention during one of my early research to examine the risks in exposure to fine-particulate air pollutants of short-term elevations. Luckily, the research failed to find any threat. Thus, a brief and occasional visit to an area where the air is terrible is not likely to trigger an episode of AFib.

However, contaminated air can cause many complications for you if care is not taken in the long run. While not everyone has the freedom to choose where they live, almost everyone can decide what they put into their bodies. Notwithstanding, the World Health Organization (WHO) recorded that more than one billion people vape or smoke tobacco products. You won't be amazed to know that people who smoke are highly at risk of having one or more episodes of atrial fibrillation in their lifetime.

This is an exception to the myriads of health-related problems caused by smoking, including emphysema and cancer.

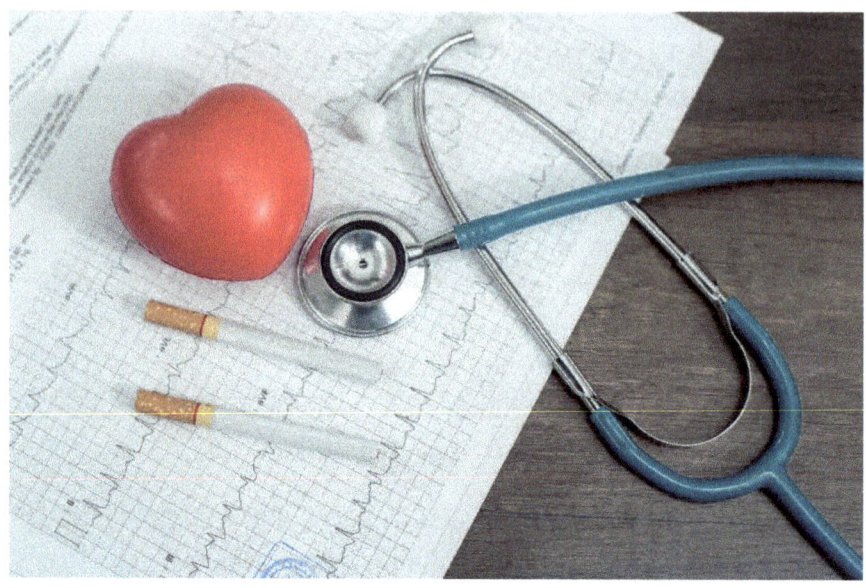

You should also know that being close to or living with a smoker can heighten your risk. Each pack of cigarettes smoked by an adult, on an average level, increases their kids' chances of having atrial fibrillation. No parents would be proud to leave this legacy behind.

You are Undergoing a lot of stress.

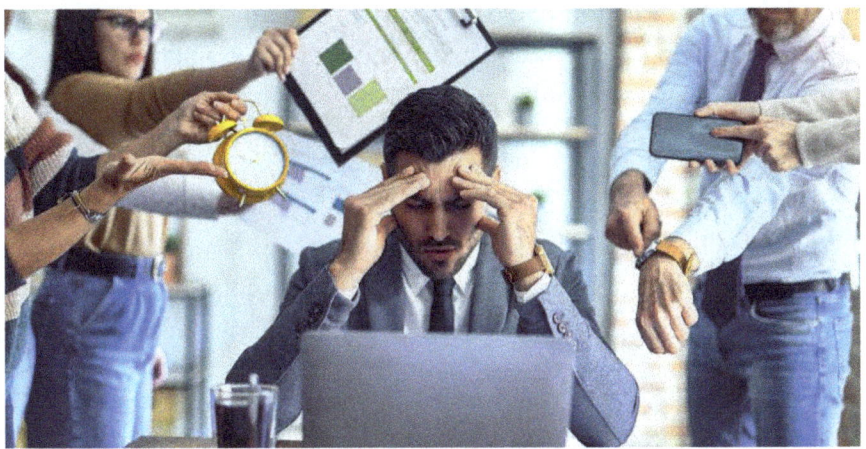

Maria was in her mid-fifties when she was diagnosed with AFib. She had lost her husband some years back, and life was now beginning to take its toll on her. A heart attack had reportedly killed her husband. It was now up to her to make things right for herself and their three kids.

At the time of her husband's death, she worked as an accountant in a mall located in the heart of the city. Since a new corporate company had now claimed the mall's ownership, she was expecting an augment in her earnings since it had been several years since she received one. This was mainly during her first kid's time in college, and the second just got admitted. "But when I mentioned a raise, they replied by telling me that my salary was way higher than what my equivalents in other malls in the city had, and for that reason I should not expect any salary increase."

To make some extra cash, Maria decided to take up a driving job in a brewery factory. "Meeting new faces was one thing I loved about the new job," she said, "but the driving part of it did not satisfy me a bit. The traffic situation could be so terrible that nothing except legs would be moving. Lots of construction work was going on at the period and what you would see every day was an assembly of big trucks, tractors, and other big conveyances, to make matters worse.

Her youngest child was also there. He had just begun middle school. Like many children in that stage of life, he found it quite challenging to get along with social groups and avoid bullies in school. The discomfort and anxiety he felt became so bad that he decided not to go to school at all for one week.

It took a concerted effort of the school principal, counsellor, a private therapist, and Maria herself to create the enabling environment he needed to go back to school.

To add insult to injury, Maria had recently been diagnosed to be hypertensive and pre-diabetic. The news of being at risk of hypertension came to her like a bolt from out of the blue.

"I didn't know things could turn around for bad that quickly, although things were pretty difficult at that time," she said.

When Maria suffered her first episode of atrial fibrillation, she was afraid, thinking it was a heart attack: the complication to which her husband had lost his life. She became more frightened because of her children. But when she discovered that she had only suffered an episode of arrhythmia, she felt relieved and calm, at least for the time being.

Long before now, psychological stress had been established to be one of the underlying factors responsible for atrial fibrillation. The risks of this are prevalent among women. However, it doesn't mean that it can't happen to men. Even cardiologists are not immune to it. This is because their line of work is often very stressful and demanding. Dr. Megan Harrison had learned this when he was just twenty-eight years old.

"I had received a call that night from our cardiac intensive care unit about a cardiac arrest," he recounted his experience in a letter he wrote to the International Journal of Cardiology. "I was forced to jump out of bed, only for me to learn later on that it was a false alert. I retired to bed and, not long after, started experiencing some palpitations. My heartbeats were fast and irregular".

An electrocardiogram (EKG) of Harrison's heart depicted AFib with a ventricular rate that exceeded 180 beats per minute. The truth is, Harrison isn't alone. A large number of doctors also fall victim to AFib. Even politicians, lawyers, accountants, athletes, CEOs, celebrities, and others have at one time or the other been confronted with AFib due to the stress they undergo.

You should ponder on this: if a single stressful incident can stimulate a young cardiologist with no previous record of heart problems, or any other medical issues for that matter, into AFib, how much more a person like Maria who was having several medical issues at the same time along with other substrate stressors.

What kind of complication can birth stress that leads to AFib? Research conducted by a group of experts in Denmark revealed that the highly tiring experience of losing a partner could increase a person's risk of having AFib for a year. Another study that looked into the issue concluded that divorced men are more susceptible to death occasioned by atrial fibrillation. Similar research has also linked AFib to work-related stress such as getting fired from work.

This research also established that people doing work with high psychological demands, usually with little or no control over the work situations are 50 percent more likely to have atrial fibrillation.

Further research has also shown that feelings of stress, anger, impatience, sadness and anxiety could increase the chance of an episode of AFib by 500 percent in a day. The reverse is the case with happiness. According to this research, a feeling of joy makes you 85 percent less vulnerable to AFib attacks.

Therefore, it is crystal clear that those who nurse deep feelings of disengagement and sadness are more prone to have AFib. Mainly, depression is not a healthy thing for the heart and the whole body.

One study revealed that incidents of depression heighten the risks of AFib by 700 percent. Luckily, this same research established that timely and quick treatment of depression could lessen the risk of AFib. However, with an increasing number of more than fifteen million Americans and hundreds of millions of people worldwide suffering from depression, the rate of depression-induced atrial fibrillation is likely to continue to soar.

But mental and emotional stress is not the only trigger that can lead to AFib. Research has revealed that episodes of atrial fibrillation can also be linked with physical stress caused by events like harmful infections, surgery, and car crashes. In the case of singular events like these, the chances of the AFib passing away when the event passes away is high and feasible.

A Breakdown of How It Happens Exactly

What exactly is going on inside the body of a person with atrial fibrillation? The answer to this question is quite challenging to come by because not everyone can relate to it. As the case may be, even medical practitioners and doctors cannot accurately describe the incidence. It remains one of the most frequently asked questions to which people need an answer.

Atrial fibrillation, as you know, is not just a disease of the heart. It only serves as a source of reference for the signs and symptoms and where they were first detected.

It is helpful to imagine one of those comical Rube Goldberg machines to understand this topic better. You are well disposed to using these things. They are some forms of contraception that are both charmingly and ridiculously constructed to connect a group of everyday items, each of them kinetically working upon the next to finish an easy task in a complex way.

A marble is dropped down a track and rolls into spring which gets sprung and hits a Matchbox car. The car goes steadily down a ramp and breaks a pinout of position. And since the pin was the one holding one end of a rope down on a pulley, and the other end was fixed to weight, the pulley is released into action.

These are the exact processes in which each of the factors mentioned above finally leads you down the atrial fibrillation path. They all combine to trigger AFib to occur.

"Have you seen a moving car suddenly lose its break before?" Fagin asked, "you know the massive speed, loss of control, and loss of direction that follow; that was exactly how it happened," he said.

A skip in a heartbeat is all that is needed for you to have atrial fibrillation.

Chapter Two: Risk Factors and Triggers

N ow that you have learned about some substrate causes of atrial fibrillation, you must get exposed to the triggers. Recall that the difference between triggers and substrate causes was explained in the previous chapter.

While substrate causes are the factors that lead to a person having atrial fibrillation, triggers, on the other hand, are things that induce specific incidents of arrhythmia. Sometimes, triggers can be so glaring, while at other times, they can be pretty tricky to decipher.

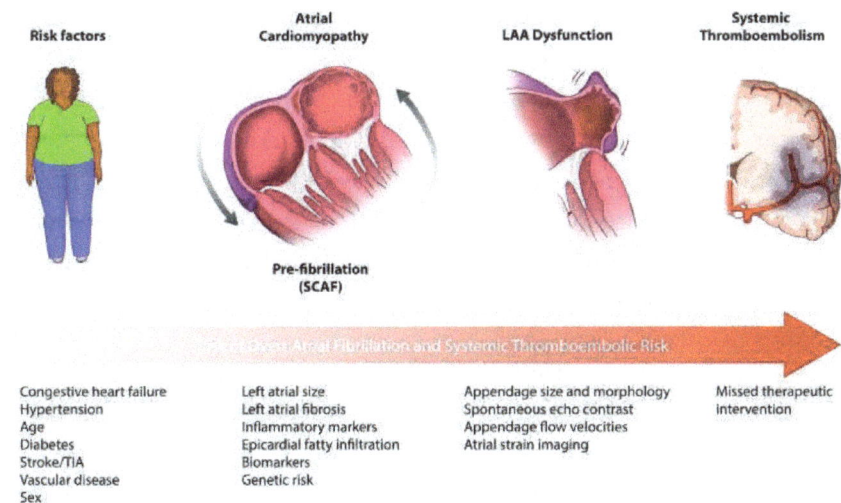

Risk factors	Atrial Cardiomyopathy	LAA Dysfunction	Systemic Thromboembolism
	Pre-fibrillation (SCAF)		
Congestive heart failure	Left atrial size	Appendage size and morphology	Missed therapeutic intervention
Hypertension	Left atrial fibrosis	Spontaneous echo contrast	
Age	Inflammatory markers	Appendage flow velocities	
Diabetes	Epicardial fatty infiltration	Atrial strain imaging	
Stroke/TIA	Biomarkers		
Vascular disease	Genetic risk		
Sex			
COPD			

Some years back, a team of researchers from the University of California in San Francisco researched to grasp better the difference in perceived triggers common with people with atrial fibrillation. They discovered in their research that people who have better and improved health always have clear motivations. At the same time, those who are less healthy may not necessarily need a catalyst to cause abnormal and irregular heartbeats (arrhythmia). They also discovered that while almost everyone has a specific trigger, some triggers are much more common than others.

The three most frequent triggers of atrial fibrillation are alcohol, caffeine, and exercise, in that order. While all of these mentioned factors are a huge part of the combined causes that make people develop atrial fibrillation, it would be very uncommon for them to be the sole cause of the condition.

But once an individual is at risk, exercise, caffeine, and alcohol can be potent inducing triggers that can push the heart out of control.

Alcohol as a trigger of atrial fibrillation should not be perceived as outrageous, should it? There are many stories shared by doctors and other medical practitioners about college students who developed AFib after drinking to stupor. Caffeine is a highly effective stimulant that can have significant effects on the heart. And since exercise is perceived as one of the most natural ways to make our body healthy and mind settled, it shouldn't be a shock to learn that if your heart is already used to beating fast, a push over the edge could give room to atrial fibrillation.

Apart from alcohol, caffeine, and exercise, another group of factors that could cause AFib to be triggered are stress or anxiety, dehydration, sleep, and large meals. That first factor is particularly an exciting thing to consider. Unlike many other factors that medical practitioners and institutions justify, stress and anxiety were validated to be great triggers of atrial fibrillation by the victims of the medical condition. Therefore, anxiety and stress could be more excellent triggers of AFib than alcohol and even exercise.

You eat large meals, don't you? And now you're surprised and want to know why food could be a potential trigger of AFib. Well, the reason isn't far-fetched. Perhaps it is due to the discovery that gastrointestinal (GI) issues are known to incite the vagus nerve, which connects the heart, gut, and brain. Although this connection has not been fully understood, research has shown that gastrointestinal (GI) diseases could be linked to AFib.

Moreover, when GI problems have been addressed, the atrial fibrillation comes down as well. Gastrointestinal (GI) triggers may be more prevalent among people as the case may be. Issues relating to stress and anxiety such as constipation, nausea, bloating, and others are possible triggers of atrial fibrillation.

Common Symptoms Associated With AFib

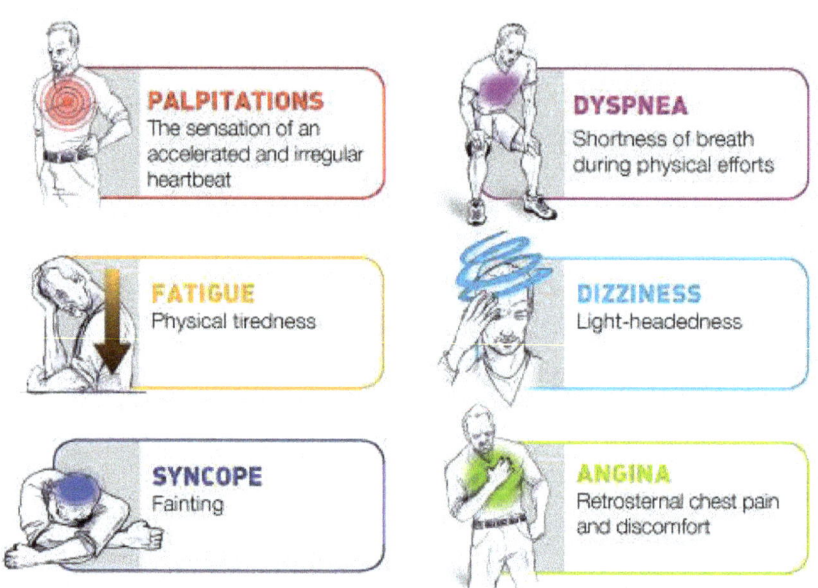

Knowledge of how atrial fibrillation disrupts blood flow through the heart and its interference with the electrical signals that help the heartbeat will help you grasp why most common symptoms that come with AFib (especially palpitations) are evident during an episode.

However, many of the victims of this phenomenon mistakenly believe that they don't experience any symptoms related to AFib because they can't feel the pulses commonly linked to this arrhythmia. Speaking from experience, the most common sign that can be associated with atrial fibrillation is not palpitations as many people suggest; instead, it is fatigue/tiredness. Behind this symptom lies a secondary symptom: shortness of breath. When considering the most suitable sign to take third place, you can then think of palpitations. And that's where all the complications come from. Since many people have reported not to have experienced palpitations with their AFib, they seldom get help when they need it.

Of course, it can be pretty challenging to associate feelings of being breathless and exhausted with a specific problem. These symptoms are geared and caused by several medications. They can also be due to irregular or no exercise at all, lack of adequate sleep, or excess weight gain. However, if you feel breathless and exhausted and can't decipher the reason you are feeling that way, you need to find out.

Nancy didn't know how to go about that initially. "Talk about recreational activities, and I would tell you the only one I enjoyed thoroughly was skiing," she recounted.

"But I couldn't keep up with it anymore. I always felt drained and weak: the way I often felt after running a race, except I wasn't running".

The reason was probably that Nancy's heart was beating faster than usual, and her body was trying to cope with it. It takes a lot of strength and energy to keep a heart super-active, the same amount of energy needed during a strenuous workout. But, just like many other people, Nancy initially perceived these symptoms as probable consequences of ageing. (This perhaps explains why when I help patients suffering from AFib return to normal heartbeats again, they often testify how much younger they felt).

Aside from these symptoms, as mentioned above, of atrial fibrillation, some other signs include dizziness, lightheadedness, and confusion. The inability to think correctly, a concept termed "brain fog," is another symptom of AFib. These symptoms do not make perfect sense until you understand the impacts of atrial fibrillation on your body. The human brain is always hungry for oxygen. Oxygen moves from one part of the body to another through the circulatory system. In the body of a healthy person, the circulatory system is well crafted to transport oxygen to the appropriate place where it is needed and at the right time. However, the reverse is the case where the organ at the center of these activities is faulty; everything else is bound to malfunction. The oxygen molecules delivered by hemoglobin (a protein constituent transported to all parts of the body by the red blood cells) may still end up at the right place, but not in the same fixed rate required by the brain to function appropriately.

All these symptoms combined are the primary reason several doctors and medical experts have mounted investigations to discover the long-term consequence of atrial fibrillation. So, what's this consequence? Brain damage. Studies conducted to validate this claim found that many of the chemical symptoms of brain damage usually heightened after a concussion, such as differentiation factor 15/stress response indicator growth, tau protein, and glial fibrillary acidic protein, are dangerously high in AFib patients. These proteins, which are conventionally increased in a bid to respond to brain injury and its barriers from other parts of the body, are released much earlier in people who have AFib; a mirror view of the harmful result of the irregular heart rhythm on the brain.

The evidence of the extent to which the brain is being damaged is not just a result of molecules moving to and fro in the body. If you want to see what the brain of people with atrial fibrillation looks likes, it is better to use an MRI. When you do this, you will see that almost half of these AFib patients have signs of brain injury, which appears as brain lesions, even if they haven't had a stroke. Those who do not suffer brain lesions caused by stroke always suffer the loss of volume, popularly referred to as "shrinkage of the brain."

Some minor patterns of brain damage known as "white matter disease" are the results of brain injury. These symptoms show damage suffered by the brain from both AFib and other medical issues like diabetes and hypertension, which are significant causes of atrial fibrillation.

It might be beneficial to explain why the rate of memory decline and dementia are relatively high among those with AFib. It is common knowledge we are all aware of since that lesions commonly found in autopsied brains of people who had dementia at the time of their death; however, where these lesions came from isn't clear to anyone. In a recent study conducted by my team of researchers, we discovered that AFib is independently linked to all forms of dementia, like Alzheimer's

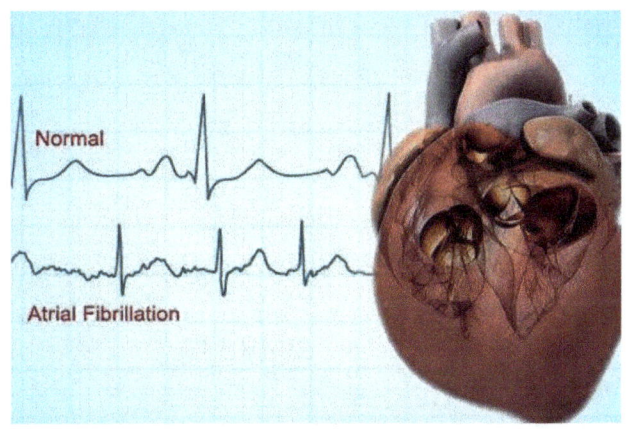

disease. Expectedly, it was found during the study that atrial fibrillation was a significant indicator that many dementia patients are at higher risks of dying. Quite unsatisfactorily, the study's findings also opined that the risk of Alzheimer's disease, especially, was drastically high among young people suffering from atrial fibrillation.

However, there is a glimmer of hope. There are many growing concerns about the phenomenon of atrial fibrillation. This has sparked a lot of interested in studying AFib. The focus of this interest is not geared towards the adverse effects of atrial fibrillation but how AFib patients can make it out of the other side with minimal consequences.

Now that you are well acquainted with the different causes of AFib, its effects on the health and functionality of the heart, and its impacts on the other organs and parts of the body and its common symptoms, you should be able to make the right health decisions.

When Should You See A Doctor?

Living with atrial fibrillation can indeed put your life on the edge. However, a special relationship with your physician can save you a lot of stress, especially when you are acquainted with when to call on him and when there is a need to go to the hospital.

As cited in the previous paragraphs, not every person living with AFib shows symptoms. They are always appalled to discover that they have arrhythmias. So, when do you call your doctor? If you have been diagnosed with AFib, you should try as much as possible to reach out to your doctor whenever you notice a symptom. This is because some of these symptoms, as the case may be, can be curatively handled. These symptoms vary from person to person, yet there are some common symptoms (highlighted in the previous section). Therefore, you need to watch out for these symptoms, and most especially stroke.

Sometimes, you do not have to wait for that long. Do you notice a flutter or quiver in the upper chamber of your heart? Are you having an abnormal and irregular electrical impulse in your core region? Do you feel like your heart is beating way too fast and beyond control? Or it feels like your heart skipped a beat? All these feelings and symptoms combined should inform you of the need to call your doctor. The reason you have to call your doctor at this time might not be so apparent to you yet. There are some symptoms of AFib that render you weak and exhausted such as dizziness and fatigue. If your atrial fibrillation finally leads to dizziness, you might find it very difficult to reach out to your doctor. The outcome of dizziness, in most cases associated with atrial fibrillation, is fainting. At this period, you are unaware of what is happening around you. Thus, it is safer and better to call your doctor's attention when the symptoms are mild.

Other symptoms associated with atrial fibrillation, as explained in the previous section, include shortness of breath, struggling to breathe, chest pain, and mental confusion. You must notify your doctor about these symptoms if you have them. If your palpitations are lasting longer than they ought to, or they are becoming more frequent than usual, you should let your doctor know.

Another set of symptoms that should make you put a call across to your doctor are signs of Congestive Heart Failure (CHF). These are also common complications of AFib because the medical condition is potent enough to weaken the heart and subject it to heart failure. Symptoms including shortness of breath and fatigue are common to CHF and AFib. This means that enough blood will not be pumped and transported to the various parts of your body. But because sufficient blood does not move at the required rate to every aspect of the body, CHF can leak fluids into other body tissues. Thus, if you notice a swelling in your ankles, feet, legs, or excess weight gain, you should endeavor to see a doctor.

CHAPTER THREE: THE FEAR

More often than not, atrial fibrillation is said to be associated with palpitations. It was a feeling described by Mike as "like comparing your heart to a washing machine into which you put a pair of boots and press the "spin" button." Others compared the condition of their heart to the sea's restive tides, which consistently go to and fro without rest. To another set of people, it was as though their hearts willingly skipped a beat.

No matter how you describe it, the bottom line is that this feeling can be seriously annoying. It can even be horrifying, especially for people who had experienced it before. People with AFib always describe their feelings as though they are "treading on eggshells"; always mindful of the fact that an unknown trigger could incite an episode of atrial fibrillation, which may require the use of cardioversions to return the earth to its regular beats. AFib occurs at anytime and anywhere. You do not risk developing AFib in one place rather than another or in one particular season or time of the year than in another. AFib does not respect time, season, or location. Thus, it can occur to you in the afternoon when you are busy cruising on the waters, or in the middle of the night when you are onboard going for a vacation in your dream city, or in a remote area where medical help is very scarce. It is the reason many AFib patients view the world as a tiny place. Therefore, they end all travels, whether long-distance or short-distance travels and stay very close to hospitals. This way, they become used to being zapped with a mini-voltage dose of electric charges (unlike what you see on the TV, the body does not jump into the air when the paddles are placed on the chest. When done in the right way, it is a painless and quick procedure void of any drama).

The issue with cardioversions is that processes do not fix anything. One can compare them to an electrical reset: capable of restarting your computer system. Research has shown that the procedures of cardioversions lead to another course of cardioversions.

Although cardioversions are said not to fix anything in the long run, they are quite indispensable in the short run, especially to people who are irrevocably committed to battling atrial fibrillation via other means. If you are often at risk of having AFib now and then, it might be pretty challenging for you to adhere strictly to the steps that will be expounded in this book. However, for many people, the thought of undergoing another process of cardioversion is often scary and frightening because they hardly know when it might be required.

"Each time my heart began beating abnormally, my mind was also not left out of the race. Even my mind would run faster than my heart", said Nancy, a competitive international skier. She was diagnosed with atrial fibrillation in her middle forties. "The fear wasn't from my head. I knew what was happening to me, and I was confident it was going to pass, but on the inside, like in my mind, the fear I might lose everything in the end often gripped me".

AFib is the result of the damage to heart cells, it's likely not new to you when you learn that majority of the deaths among AFib patients are linked to cardiovascular issues, with heart failure responsible for no less than half of those deaths.

It makes a lot of sense, doesn't it? Heart failure happens when the lower chambers of the heart, called ventricles, become too stiff or too weak, thereby making it hard for them to fill with blood as the heartbeats. So, what are the ventricles filled with? Of course, the atria, where atrial fibrillation happens.

Heart failure, as explained earlier, is occasioned when the heart becomes too stiffened and too weakened. It sure sounds like something you've heard or learned about. However, the same conditions that stimulate atrial fibrosis can also result in the remodeling of the ventricles and fibrosis of the ventricles, which can intimately cause the failure of the heart.

Death caused by heart failure can be a terrible experience, with pain that moves around every part of the body (from head to toe). So also is the persistent struggle for breath, the inability of the body to retain fluids, and in some very horrible situations, a final very few moments in panic and fear of what their fate would be. Indeed, if all that AFib could be potent enough to incite were increased risk of heart failure, then it would be sufficient to use everything at one's disposal to fight against it. But there is a piece of good news. Studies have found out that if AFib could be the potential cause of heart failure, then attempts to eliminate AFib can also eliminate the risks of heart failure. Unfortunately, the not-so-good news is that heart failure cannot be said to be the only problem caused by AFib that causes the death of the patients in the end. There are a lot more.

Let's take a look at the second cause of death of people with AFib: infection. That doesn't make sense?

The association between atrial fibrillation and infections is not strictly causal. People who are not healthy, in some way, are likely to be more susceptible to infections.

The ironic part of it is that people who, for one reason or the other, stay around the vicinity of hospitals are also more vulnerable to developing a health-related infection. The healthcare statistics released in the United States showed that about 100,000 people lose their lives each year due to diseases gotten from medical treatment. Looking vividly at this and considering the figures more carefully, it is evident that this is nearly three times the number of people who lose their lives in motor vehicle accidents every year. Having atrial fibrillation increases your risk of hospitalization, which exposes you to contracting different infections while in a healthcare facility.

There may be a direct association between atrial fibrillation and infections, to be candid. AFib is a disease induced by damaged cells, and the immune system (the system in the human body that fights against infections) treats damaged cells in a similar way it treats pathogens and irritants-with inflammation. For instance, a study showed that the gastrointestinal (GI) tract, when infected by Helicobacter pylori (a type of bacterium), results in high rates of AFib and increased immune or inflammatory response.

The collective immune response referred to as inflammation, has several benefits. Without it, damaged cells and tissues can't be healed, neither can infections be controlled. However, when it occurs over and over again, it can spell a lot of trouble. That is especially true whenever diseases are concerned. The problem arises when the immune system exhausts all its energy in fighting against atrial fibrillation: What will it fight against infectious pathogens and irritants? Hence, chronic inflammation can be directly linked to an increased risk of AFib.

The talks about the fears of atrial fibrillation cannot be completed without mentioning stroke, a life-threatening medical condition that often results in death.

Strokes are a medical condition characterized by a cut-off in the pathways of the free flow of blood to the brain. This cut-off causes the downstream parts of the brain to die within seconds.

Permit me to take you down memory lane by reminding you of the world's most famous case of an AFib-connected stroke which happened on the 18th of April, 1994. On that faithful day, Richard Nixon, a former president of the United States, while sitting at the table to eat dinner after a long day of preparation for a speech, had a terrible stroke from an AFib-incited blood clot. Almost immediately, the right side of his body became paralyzed, and he couldn't speak anymore. And although he was instantaneously rushed to the Cornell Medical Center (New York Hospital) in New York City, he couldn't be saved by some of the best doctors in the world. Four days later, his death was announced. What he left behind was a vital warning for people with atrial fibrillation and a complicated legacy.

Why are incidents of stroke common with AFib patients? The severe electrical damage in the atria results in loss of pumping. The outcome of this is a lack of blood flow and dormant blood clots, particularly in the left atrial appendage. When these blood clots get broken off and enter into the bloodstream, they are like weapons sent to any part of the body to wreak great havoc. Clots that head to the legs, kidneys, or gut can leave indelible marks of destruction behind. But when clots head to the brain, leading to a stroke, the effect is within seconds, devastating, and usually deadly.

So, what exactly happens during a stroke? Generally, during a stroke, the brain is deprived of nutrients and oxygen, which leads to the brain cells' death almost immediately. You will also remember that atrial fibrillation is often linked to high blood pressure. That's the worst because continuous high blood pressure can harm arteries in the brain even before the AFib clot arrives. Given all these reasons and facts, atrial fibrillation has been linked to increasing the risk of stroke by five times. Of course, those risks aren't the same. Several factors are militating against them—the ruse with age and other challenging medical situations. Even among people with AFib who are relatively healthy and young, there is no safe route from a stroke. Strokes in people with AFib that do not result in death always have worse disabilities than strokes induced by other factors. Even the most minimal event of stroke can cause dementia and impaired cognition.

Of course, the fear of atrial fibrillation isn't always about death. It's often more of feelings of its impacts on our individual lives; in such a way that it makes many people feel like the end wouldn't be so bad after all.

Complications and Preventions

There are a large number of complications surrounding the phenomenon of atrial fibrillation. These complications more often than not induce several questions in the mind of many people, including those who have not been diagnosed with atrial fibrillation. So, what are some of these complicated questions?

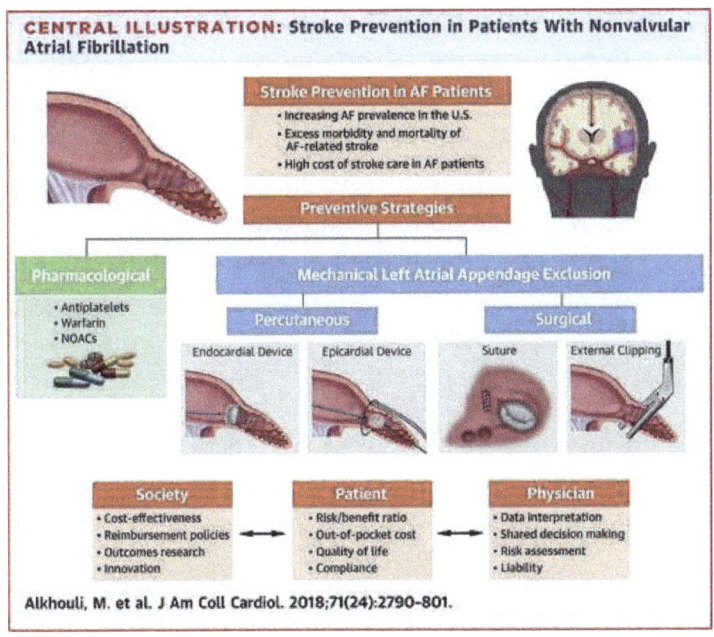

CENTRAL ILLUSTRATION: Stroke Prevention in Patients With Nonvalvular Atrial Fibrillation

Alkhouli, M. et al. J Am Coll Cardiol. 2018;71(24):2790-801.

What if I'm Not Sure I have Atrial Fibrillation?

Although this is not common, you should know that palpitations don't occur to people the same way. For some individuals, pulses can come in the form of fluttering. As a result of this, many people often confuse atrial fibrillation for atrial flutter, a type of arrhythmia that occurs in the upper chamber of the heart. So, what is the fundamental difference between the two? While AFib is characterized by a fast and irregular heartbeat, atrial flutter, on the other hand, involves a quick and regular rhythm.

The fact that atrial flutter includes a fast and regular rhythm doesn't mean that it doesn't have any adverse effect. Worse still, atrial flutter can result in the wrong things familiar with atrial fibrillation, such as heart failure, strokes, and the like. Yes, both of them also have similar triggers. Also, whatever treatment is recommended for atrial fibrillation can treat atrial flutter. Thus, while you will likely see "AFib" on every page of this book, have it in mind that the prevention techniques can be used to address these two types of arrhythmias.

Do I Have To Take The Risk?

Well, atrial fibrillation itself is a risk, and if you are not ready to fight it back, you might be left in the lurch. On the other hand, suppose you have been diagnosed with AFib, and you intend to stick to the conventional means of using medications. In that case, you might be subjecting yourself to a much greater risk induced by increasingly debilitating symptoms. However, if you choose to follow the tricks and steps that are explained in this book, you will likely, and most certainly, improve the quality of your health and life.

Does this apply to only young people?

The first question you have to answer is that "what is your definition of young?" Do you mean someone in his early thirties or someone in her early eighties? The phenomenon of atrial fibrillation has no regard for age. It is common in both the young and the old. Although the old are more vulnerable to fall victim to it due to some underlying factors to which they are likely to be susceptible due to their age. Yet, cases of AFib have increasingly become popular among young people in recent years. Thus, no one is exempted from the problem.

In this same vein, this book is helpful to both the young and the old. Even those in their late eighties have used tips gathered from this book to fight against AFib by getting off medications, taking transformational steps, and making rational lifestyle decisions that will always help them stay healthy.

Why Do I Need My Doctor?

Can you handle your sickness all alone? Not to talk of a medical condition as critical as atrial fibrillation. Perhaps you should know that this is more complicated than what you think. Maybe you haven't ever experienced it before or are not close to someone who had it. It isn't an attempt to make you afraid. You can know that you are battling a severe medical condition with heart failure and strokes as symptoms. What could be more devastating? Therefore, you seriously need the attention of a doctor.

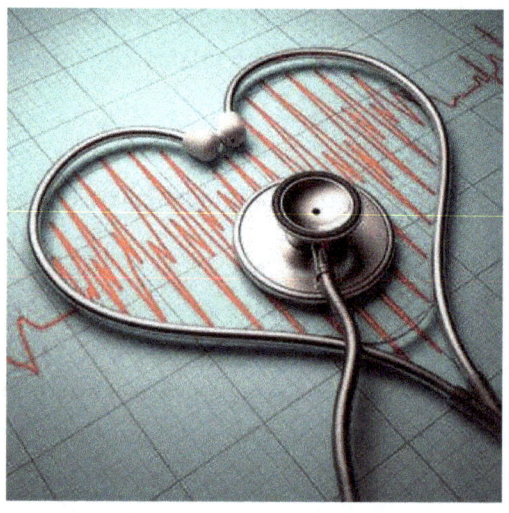

Also, if you have ever been diagnosed with atrial fibrillation, it is a sign that you need a doctor. Although some physicians offer little or no hope of recovery from AFib, that doesn't mean they don't want you to be well. Also, don't see this book as the perfect replacement for your doctor. A doctor is indispensable. The focus of this piece is to educate and make you well-informed about AFib. If you do not have a doctor at your disposal, what you will learn in this book is why you need a doctor to see you through the process. Don't make things complicated for yourself. You'll need an electrophysiologist: a physician who specializes in the care of arrhythmias. They will help you understand what your heart is trying to tell you at every point in time.

Does It Mean That I Have To Undergo Surgery?

Don't get it all muddled up. The surgical procedure used in this regard is popularly known as ablation. It involves moving a thin, flexible tube through the blood vessels into a patient's heart, where one of many techniques is used to amend the irregular electrical pathways that cause atrial fibrillation. Although these surgical procedures are essential to the treatment of AFib, they are not a foregone alternative. Even without these procedures, a good number of people with AFib have put their life back on track.

Do I Have To Be Acquainted With Technology?

Rather than technology, atrial fibrillation is a natural occurrence. Although this is often a result of irregular and abnormal electrical shifts, it has little or no connection with technology. Instead, impulses generate electrical changes in this regard.

Getting yourself acquainted with technological devices of any kind as far as this is concerned I'd not find necessary. What you need is the ability to collect some simple data about your health and living standards. This encompasses tracking your workout, meals, and a whole lot of other factors that have been said to cause and trigger atrial fibrillation.

Interestingly, science and technology have done more good in recent times than fighting health-related issues that come with AFib.

With the aid of this duo, consumer technologies that can quickly detect risks of having an atrial fibrillation event before it rears its ugly head have been devised. Many smart watches can help you see a sign of potential atrial fibrillation even before an episode of arrhythmia happens. These "wearable" devices have made it possible, even without the help of doctors, for people to be well informed about their medical condition. It has become a popular subject of discussion in public as a result of these devices. They have also contributed immensely to the quick diagnosis of atrial fibrillation.

One of such smart watches is an EKG-enabled smart watch. So yes, an EKG-enabled smart watch can help you immensely.

If you look vividly at some of the causes of atrial fibrillation, it is effortless to say that avoiding these substrate causes is the best way to prevent the occurrence of AFib. For easy reference, you can prevent atrial fibrillation by doing the following:

- Get enough sleep. You must ensure that you go to bed as and at when due.
- Engage in exercise. The benefit of doing exercise is vast. If you want to reduce the risk of having AFib, you should embrace daily and consistent workouts.
- Take good care of your health as you age. If you know you are not on the good side of age anymore, you should seek medical advice on how to stay healthy.
- Watch your diet. Processed and fast foods increase your chances of developing atrial fibrillation by five times. Choose more plant-based meals.
- Avoid taking energy drinks. These drinks are known to contain a lot of caffeine which increases your chances of having AFib. Therefore, you have to prevent it by avoiding energy drinks.

- Like energy drinks, alcohol is also detrimental to your health and makes you even more susceptible to having AFib. So cut down your consumption of alcohol.
- Do you smoke, or you live in a highly polluted environment? You have to quit smoking if you don't want atrial fibrillation. Watch out for the health status of your environment; make sure that factors that can make you vulnerable to AFib are gotten rid of.
- If you have been diagnosed with any heart problem before, ensure that you treat it very well to prevent it from leading to atrial fibrillation.
- If yours is a result of the genetic components passed down to you by your parents, you should make your doctor your best friend. He will help in that regard.
- Take good care of your blood pressure. A high level of blood pressure heightens your risk of having AFib, so you can do yourself a lot of good by watching out for it.
- Do you just take drugs without thinking about the effects and implications that these drugs are likely to have on you and your health? You shouldn't do that anymore. Some medications you are using, perhaps for other medical conditions you are battling with, may be exposing you to atrial fibrillation. Thus, don't use drugs without the full knowledge and consent of your doctor.
- Supplements and vitamins can be responsible for AFib, so endeavour to tell your doctor about the supplements and vitamins you are using.
- You are probably too engaged in many activities. As a result, you end up stressed each night. By doing this every day, you are increasing your chances of having AFib. So, if you don't want to have AFib, you have to have some rest.

- Make sure that your thyroid hormone level is balanced. The story of your body Vitamin D is vital as well. Take those into consideration.
- Reduce the rate at which you consume sugar.

Conclusion – Part 1

The various attributes and factors discussed in this part are only familiar to very few people. However, the truth is that many people who have fallen victim to atrial fibrillation today are more likely to be doing at least one or more of the substrate causes of AFib. It's also highly scarce to come across an atrial fibrillation patient who does not have many of these factors in their lives.

Whether or not such a condition is due to genetic or biological makeup, engaging other factors is all that is needed to incite an otherwise healthy individual into a harmful state of arrhythmias.

But as clear as these descriptions are, these factors can lead to other health conditions. Atrial fibrillation happens by chance to be the one that occurs first. In comparison to a coal mine, AFib can be said to be the canary. And just like the young yellow bird that coalminers take along with them to deep underground to detect the presence of deadly gases, AFib could be a condition that benefits your life than harms it. As much as you are ready and willing to take advantage of transformational procedures and make rational decisions that will help you live a healthy life, AFib can be very treatable.

Although, a similar thing can't be said about stroke. It is the most life-threatening complication of atrial fibrillation. While the first occurrence of atrial fibrillation may not necessarily mean the end for you, the same cannot be said about stroke. Stroke is often a final death experience for hundreds of thousands of people across the world.

Also, a similar thing cannot be said about other health complications like dementia, Alzheimer's disease, and vascular infections. Research has further proven that all those infections, which have little or no chance to be reversed, are independently connected to AFib.

Studies have revealed that atrial fibrillation is a "risk indicator" for future cancer occurrence, which eventually kills about half of its victims. Atrial fibrillation has also been linked with chronic kidney infections, heart failure, venous thromboembolism, and heart attack. This was made possible through peer-reviewed research.

So, what AFib does, is offer you the privilege to get ahead of all these hurdles. To hear and heed the clarion call. To recognize that something is wrong somewhere.

A Checklist of AFib Substrate Causes

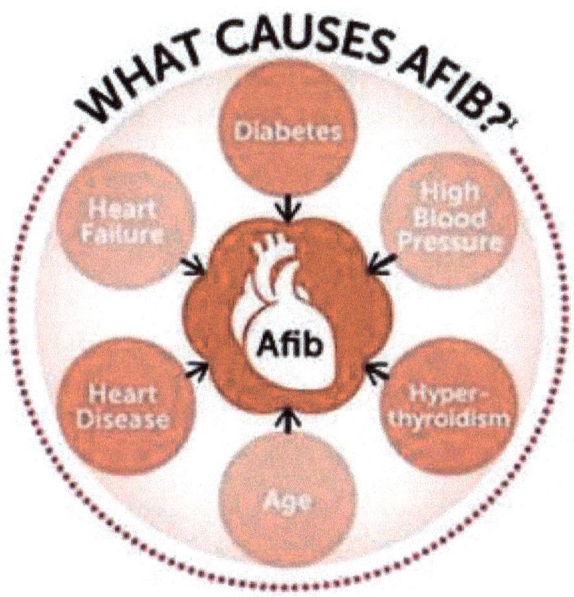

This is not a complete list of all the substrate causes of atrial fibrillation. Also, none of these causes validates that you are at risk of AFib, although there might be chances. The more the number of factors you tick, the more effort you will apply to put your atrial fibrillation to remission. No matter the number of these factors you find in yourself, don't be discouraged; there's undoubtedly someone else somewhere who's picking up from where you stopped.

Check the causes that may apply to you.

Known or possible genetic Vulnerability

- ✓ You or any member of your family developed atrial fibrillation before the age of forty-five.
- ✓ A genetic diagnosis has confirmed a mutation in some genes linked with AFib
- ✓ A member of your family have atrial fibrillation

Other Current or Former Heart Complications

- ✓ Heart failure
- ✓ Heart Blockage
- ✓ Heart valve issues
- ✓ Heart attack

Blood Pressure

- ✓ Over 130/80

Age

- ✓ Over the age of ninety
- ✓ Over the age of eighty
- ✓ Over the age of seventh
- ✓ Over the age of sixty
- ✓ Over the age of fifty

Medications and other Drugs

✓ Non-steroidal anti-inflammatory drugs (naproxen, ibuprofen, and others)
✓ Steroids
✓ Proton-pump inhibitors (Protonix, Prevacid, Prilosec, and others)
✓ Diuretics
✓ THC/Marijuana
✓ Anti-arrhythmics
✓ Stimulants
✓ Thyroid hormone

Processed Carbohydrates and Sugar

✓ Regular consumption of processed carbohydrates
✓ Regular consumption of sugar

Exercise

✓ Endurance sports and activities
✓ Little or no exercise program

Sleep

✓ Sleep apnea
✓ Less or more than eight to nine hours of sleep per night

Alcohol and/or Energy Drinks

- ✓ Consumption of alcohol
- ✓ Consumption of energy drinks

Pollution and Smoking

- ✓ Poor quality of air in your immediate environment
- ✓ Smoking and any other use of tobacco

Emotional and Mental Stress

- ✓ Impatience
- ✓ Anxiety
- ✓ Stress
- ✓ Sadness
- ✓ Anger
- ✓ Depression

INTRODUCTION – PART 2

Understanding Medication

Something was out of place. Flora is a forty-seven-year-old project supervisor in a nursing school but couldn't even decipher what it was. She had visited her doctor after suffering an attack of atrial fibrillation earlier that day. She was now on her way home.

"It was such an ugly experience", she recalled "it was just some minutes past 4 AM when it all began. I thought that was going to be the end. My heartbeat rose within seconds and was beating faster than it ought to. Until then, I never knew that the heart could beat at such a fast rate. And then, all by itself, it stopped", she added.

"When I got to the emergency room, I met a couple of doctors there".

"They advised me to get in touch with my primary care physician. And just immediately, I made it straight to my doctor's office. He gave me a pleasant reception perhaps because he had not seen me in ages", she explained further.

But the warm reception wasn't all that she wanted. And because that wasn't all she wanted, she felt somewhat disappointed.

"I expected a list of things to do, some procedures, just some random stuff to ease myself off the stress".

"But he just told me there's nothing much he can do and that it's going to keep getting worse as I age. He added that being diagnosed with high blood pressure is a complication. But he had some prescriptions to give me; anyways."

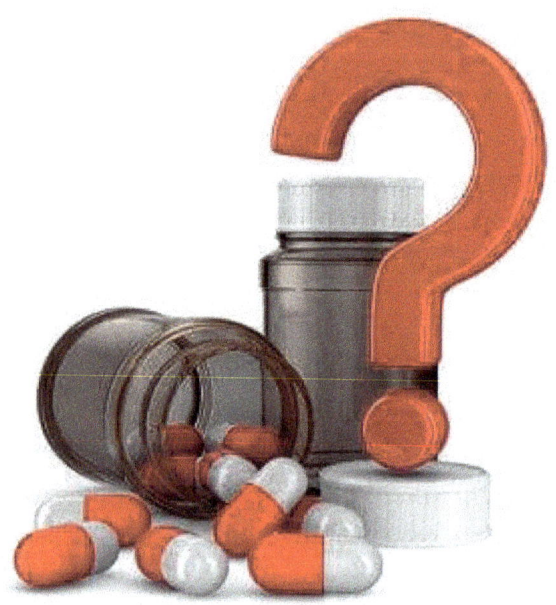

Flora had a lot of questions she wanted to ask him but didn't realize this until she was already driving home "Just like when you wake up from your slumber, I thought, 'this can't be everything, there's surely going to be another way around it'" she said.

Well, Flora's instinct was correct after all. But her experience with her doctor wasn't unexpected. For all of the triggers and reasons discussed in the first part of this book, and several others, a large number of doctors still treat people suffering from atrial fibrillation as victims of an unavoidable condition that deteriorates over time.

More often than not, there is a slowdown in diagnoses, particularly if you have your first attack of atrial fibrillation. Among the very few diagnosed individuals, just one or two of them will proceed to a cardiologist for stress and fatigue testing. As indispensable as cardiac electrophysiologist are in this case, not too many people will make it to them. What's worse than this? As a result of the failure to undergo these vital diagnoses and fresh episodes of AFib each passing day, the condition is likely to become harder and harder to solve or treat. Thus, if you do not acquaint yourself with sufficient knowledge and make up your mind to make a lasting resolution, there are good chances that you will just be prescribed drugs to thin your blood and slow your heart, then be asked to go home like Flora.

The truth is, these medications can't be termed "bad". Also, the doctors who advise their patients to tread this path of using drugs aren't terrible people who are trying to subject their patients to a life of mystery and dilemma. Their intention is quite clear. And this healthy and friendly intention of theirs is one backed up by several years of studies and research that reveal that people who are not on the good side of age (say age sixty-five and above) are more at risk of suffering atrial fibrillation. Those who fail to perform diagnosis for their patients when they suffer an episode of AFib should not be seen as evil because not every incident of atrial fibrillation comes with an episode of arrhythmia. That is because even the rumor that there's usually a drop-off of about 20 to 30 per cent in cardiac performance associated with AFib due to the age factor is valid since most aged people are known to be immobile. Thus, the prescription of medication isn't wrong.

Medication isn't harmful. Contrarily, an overdependence on drugs might not give you the desired result you seek. So, you want to know why precisely many doctors prescribe medication for AFib patients. Their prescriptions are based on the research that supports the opinion that people with AFib can genuinely be made to feel "better" when they are offered medications that will slow their heartbeats down. Moreover, by slowing the heart down, these medications may prevent you from having heart failure. There is also evidence that blood thinners, to a large extent, reduce the risk of having a stroke. These are treatments that can give you hope.

Many physicians are yet to have a deep understanding of that making atrial fibrillation treatable in the short run, without efforts to achieve a long-term good health goal, will eventually leave the patient(s) in the lurch because atrial fibrillation is a battle against time. One episode of AFib leads to another, and in some cases can beget other health hazards, doctors have a short space of time during which their patients' heart will adequately respond to treatment, and as guaranteed by research, put the condition into remission. So, how long is your window of opportunity? Well, that's different for each person. If what you are suffering from is a once-in-a-while episode of AFib that corrects itself, that time could be a range of years spanning to as much as ten years (for people with familial AFib and otherwise stable heart). However, if your AFib does not correct itself, then the time at your disposal might not be up to a year- that's if it's not even a couple of months.

There's also another reason many physicians are yet to embrace a positive view of this condition. There's little peer-reviewed research (the type of research that patients want doctors to adhere strictly to while administering drugs) showing that patients can do without medications. It indicates that they can live a better and improved life after an AFib experience and that atrial fibrillation can be put to remission. To be sure, there are several research and studies of this type (peer-reviewed research) that support these ideas. However, the problem is that these studies and research are built up against years of relative inaction and previous thoughts and have been delayed to affect the mainstream medical perception positively.

Change is the only constant thing in life, and it is in progress as far as this phenomenon is concerned. At conferences organized to look into atrial fibrillation, researchers and physicians from all parts of the world made revelations vital to creating an AFib-free world. Not too many of these physicians believe this is possible to achieve. Many of them support the idea that making life-changing decisions, particularly those that affect people's lifestyle and ways of living, can be pretty challenging to make. The controversies surrounding the genetic causes of atrial fibrillation and the lack of sufficient enlightened EPs for each person in the world suffering from atrial fibrillation further reiterate their claim. The good news is that these conferences chaired by pessimistic doctors and researchers have turned around to accommodate optimism in recent years. There's true light at the end of the tunnel.

There are myriads of medications from which your doctor can decide to prescribe one or more for you. Having a good understanding of what these medications do will help you a lot. These medications come with benefits as well as side effects. Some medicines that are often used in treating atrial fibrillation include the following:

Antiarrhythmic Medications

These medications are popularly referred to as "the rhythm keepers" because they are specially designed to ensure that your heart is kept in rhythm. There aren't many types of these medications. Also, because these medications have many side effects attached to them, you hardly find them in most pharmaceutical stores. As mentioned earlier, antiarrhythmic can only keep your heart in rhythm for one year. If it's more than that, its chance of being effective is fifty-fifty. One adverse side effect that is known about these drugs is cardiac arrest.

No medication comes without having one or more side effects. And that's the truth. Even for any drug to be potent enough to repair the damage done by atrial fibrillation, such medication must have significant impacts on the whole parts of the body. How great an impact? You will know it takes many skills and mental capacity for an electrician to wire a house. A single mistake in wiring can make the house a mess. The human body is more intricate than a house and far more valuable. When there is a mess in how the body cells interact and connect with the electrical charges that usually move in every part of the body, then there are tendencies of being at risk of not just AFib but also other medical complications.

Some common examples of antiarrhythmic medications are amiodarone, sotalol, flecainide, dofetilide, propafenone, and dronedarone. These aren't the only kinds of antiarrhythmic drugs, but they are the commonest. Irrespective of any of these medications you are trying to take, or probably you have been advised to use, or you are already using, there are certain things you need to understand.

If one type of antiarrhythmic fails to address the problem, it is implausible for the other types to work. The only exception to this assertion is amiodarone.

Using an antiarrhythmic to fight against any medical condition (not just atrial fibrillation in this case) is likely to shorten your life. So, if you are not careful enough while using these drugs, your life expectancy is expected to be affected.

As a result of the fact that you are using these medications to improve your health, you must endeavor to look at the bright side and not the side effects attached to them.

Antiarrhythmics are known to have a short period of effectiveness. As cited earlier, these medications afford you a fifty-fifty chance of putting your heart in rhythm.

The Rate Controllers

What is the job of these medications? They slow your heart down. The truth is, if your heart is beating so fast, let's say at the rate of 150 beats per minute, then gradually reducing it is better. Whether your heart is in an active state of atrial fibrillation or not, rate controllers slow the heart down no matter what. The consequence is bradycardia: a medical condition in which the heart is too slow to pump and transport blood rich in oxygen to the various parts of the body. This condition is prevalent in older people who are either on the edge of fainting or even fainting due to heart rates of less than forty-five beats per minute. Hence, the advice is always to ensure that you have a smartwatch or any other device to monitor and control your heart rate if you are on any rate controllers.

Rate controllers, like antiarrhythmics, have a purpose in the human body. Apart from making you feel "better" even when you have AFib, they also help you curtail the risks of heart failure when your heartbeats rise during an episode of AFib. Our hearts can't keep running for seven days in a week and twenty-four hours each day and continue working correctly. So, what quantity of rate controllers is required to keep the body and mind in good shape?

As much as you do not have any symptoms related to AFib, research reveals that an atrial fibrillation heart rate of fewer than 110 beats each minute is the safest. Rate controllers can achieve that if used under the right conditions.

The popular types of rate controllers are beta-blockers, digoxin, and calcium channel inhibitors. Unfortunately, some of the side effects associated with antiarrhythmics apply to rate controllers as well. Therefore, if you are using a combination of antiarrhythmic and rate controllers, your heartbeat rate might drop to a relatively low point that you can faint due to lack of sufficient oxygen to your brain or develop relatively low blood pressure. You are likely to experience this if you are not on the good side of age.

If you are taking any of these rate controllers, or it has been prescribed for you, there are certain things you should know. Some of these things are:

Your heart may be kept out of rhythm due to the low heartbeat rate.

When it comes to safety, they are relatively safer than antiarrhythmic.

Blood Thinners

Because AFib increases the risks of a stroke, physicians are often quick to prescribe an anticoagulant. These drugs also referred to as blood thinners; help prevent the formation of clots inside the heart. These are the keepers of the flow of blood in the heart. The less likely it is for a blood clot to be formed in the left atrial appendage, which often takes place when the upper parts of the heart stop beating during an AFib attack, the less likely it is for a clot to break off, leading to short supply of blood and inadequate supply of oxygen to the brain and other organs in the body.

For several years, aspirin was thought to be protective against strokes suffered from atrial fibrillation. But as we would have it, they discovered that the cheap and common remedy to render little or no help. While you might be thinking that the risk of suffering a stroke can be reduced by simply adhering to taking an aspirin a day, a recent study has shown that aspirin, even in individuals who have a lower risk of having atrial fibrillation, actually doesn't work in this regard. Instead, what it does is that it increases the risk of AFib patients suffering devastating internal bleeding.

Although it is pretty essential to prevent AFib strokes, when the natural blood clotting ability of the body is blocked, you are likely to be interfering with a process that is vital to your being alive. But, since a stroke isn't what anyone desires, blood thinners represent another pharmaceutical compromise. Because of the enormous risks attached to using these medications, there's a pressing need for both physicians and patients to take a shared decision before they are prescribed.

For individuals whose atrial fibrillation episodes last for more than forty-eight hours and require cardioversion, the choice is relatively easy to make: you should be on an anticoagulant for a minimum of a month. There's nothing magical about the forty-eight-hour principle; it is a conservative or rough estimate of how long the formation of a blood clot is going to take to develop in the left atrial appendage. According to some research, these blood clots can be formed in twenty-four hours or less, or even as minimal as seven minutes. For every other person, the decision to use an anticoagulant should be made after a thoughtful and thorough evaluation of the risks attached has been done.

Some common examples of blood thinners or anticoagulants are warfarin, Xarelto, savaysa, Pradaxa, and apixaban. The vital thing to grasp is that the benefit-vs-risk balance between internal bleeding and stroke is often delicate and can be worsened if you decide to add another medication (let's take, for instance, heart failure medications) to these blood thinners. Take note that:

All blood thinners thin the blood to significantly reduce the risk of a stroke caused by a blood clot.

Anticoagulants generally increase the risk of internal bleeding.

Medications for Heart Failure

The association between heart failure and atrial fibrillation is so deep that experts and researchers described the two diseases as "a dual epidemic". A study conducted by Danish health scientists discovered that about 10 per cent of patients suffering from heart failure have or will have AFib within three and a half years. Heart failure doesn't mean that your heart has finally stopped working; if that were the case, medications wouldn't have been necessary.

What happens during heart failure is the inability of the heart ventricles to contract as vigorously as it ought to or fill as adequately as it should. Regardless of atrial fibrillation, this condition is expected to get harder and harder to correct if nothing is done to get it treated. So, heart failure can gradually lead to a heart that will stop working.

Even heart failure is likely to be triggered by a few days of the heart beating vigorously in active atrial fibrillation. Contrarily, the heart failure can be put into remission after a few months of regular sinus rhythm if the condition had been induced only by atrial fibrillation. Irrespective of the state of things, if you have been diagnosed with heart failure and AFib or a low ejection fraction, your doctor can be expected to recommend that you take more medications such as angiotensin-receptor neprilysin inhibitors (ARNIs). He can also suggest a fusion of two blood pressure-lowering peptides that reduce the blood volume, angiotensin-converting enzymes (ACE) inhibitors that dilate blood vessels and decrease blood pressure. Other medications such as angiotensin receptor blockers (ARBs) which reflex the arteries and veins for a similar purpose as ACE and Beta-blockers, which reduce pumping force and heart rate and Diuretics used to get rid of excess fluid retained from heart failure, and other medications.

Supplements

Although these are not often perceived as drugs, since they perform roles similar to those performed by drugs, their vitality can't be underestimated. Supplements include minerals, vitamins, chemicals, and herbs that play critical roles in an individual's health. The problem is that these supplements are yet to undergo the rigorous examination of pharmaceuticals. For AFib supplements, none are FDA approved. Even the supplement industry is such a one that is not regulated; thus, it can be pretty hard to know if you are getting the supplements of your choice, in the desired quantity, and void of any toxic elements. Hence, if you choose to use supplements, you should know that the decision is at your own risk, and the need for you to first discuss it with your cardiologist cannot be over-emphasized.

Some might rise to oppose the notion that since supplements aren't tested or regulated, physicians should not even make mention of them. That can be inappropriate. Whatever the case, people with atrial fibrillation are significantly turning to these chemicals for help. There are good chances of improvements if used in the correct quantity and for the right reason.

Some examples of these supplements are magnesium, potassium, nattokinase, fish oil, Vitamin D, L-carnitine, coenzyme Q10, vitamin K2, CBD oil, hawthorn, and several others. So, what are the purposes of these supplements in the human body? Let's take a quick look at them below.

- **Potassium:** This supplement helps with atrial fibrillation and palpitations. It has a minimal therapeutic window. But a high level of potassium comes with some risks.

- **Magnesium:** This element helps with palpitations, anxiety, sleep, and AFib. It comes with a bit of risk.

- **Vitamin D:** Your risk of AFib decreases with a low level of Vitamin D in the body. Ensure to consult your doctor to know if the status of this vitamin is in the normal range and quantity. Having too much of this supplement may increase your risk of AFib.

- **Fish oil:** Recent research hasn't revealed any potential benefit. However, it is suitable for increased triglycerides and has some blood-thinning impacts. If you take this supplement as directed by your doctor, you are not likely to suffer any risk.

- **Nattokinase:** It is the most popular natural anticoagulant. It is yet to be linked to atrial fibrillation. It is also not powerful to prevent strokes that come with AFib. If you combine this supplement with other medications, such as strong blood thinners, you will likely suffer bleeding.

- **L-carnitine:** It can reduce AFib. It may also aggravate arterial heart blockages and AFib via TMAO production. Hence, it is safer to avoid using it.

- **Coenzyme Q10:** It is a joint supplement of the heart. It can help correct heart failure. People who are undergoing cholesterol-lowering statins can use it as well. If taken as directed, you won't experience any adverse side effects.

- **Vitamin K2:** This can help prevent arterial calcification, especially in the heart, and safeguard the health of the body bones. If you are already taking warfarin, then this is not necessary. If taken as directed, you won't have any adverse effects.

- **CBD Oil:** Although this has not been studied to have any association with atrial fibrillation, it has been of help to AFib patients. It helps address health issues such as hypertension and diabetes. One common side effect is the damage of the liver. You can avoid using it until research has proven it to help address AFib.

- **Hawthorn:** It can help in the treatment of heart failure. It is also known to alter the channels of potassium in the heart with unknown effects. Until more research has been carried out on it, you should avoid using it.

CHAPTER ONE

BIOMARKER MONITORING: WHAT YOUR BODY IS TELLING YOU

I f you were looking for a certified nurse with several years of experience in the medical field, then Stella was one. She had spent years working in the intensive care unit of a big hospital. So, the first time she had an episode of atrial fibrillation, she couldn't help but laugh at the situation. It was a ridiculous experience for her.

There she was that evening with relatives and friends celebrating one of her kid's birthdays. She began to feel somewhat unwell. She reached out for a finger oximeter, a medical device that measures pulse rate and oxygen saturation in the blood. Her heartbeats were becoming abnormal. She was having 160 beats per minute.

That was the first time she had AFib, and perhaps that wouldn't be the last. Every new month after the first episode came with a fresh attack. The seizures kept coming and coming. Instead of mitigating, they became more constant and harmful. And then she soon had the worst nightmare of her life. She was on her way to the hospital where she worked that faithful day when it all started.

"I pushed myself harder to reach the gate of the hospital", she said. "My pulse rate had increased like the wildfire of California, and it was now challenging for me to breathe".

She was shaking, sweating, nauseating, and feeling dizzy. Her heart, from 180 beats per minute, was heading towards 200. It continued to 220, and it didn't stop there. It reached 240.

"This is it", she had thought as she recalled her experience. "This is going to be the end. My heart will stop now, and that's all for me".

Indeed, Stella was in bad condition, a terrible condition, but she sailed through and got the help and knowledge she needed to save her own life. She was able to follow through the processes and thus, put her AFib into total remission. To achieve that, Stella had to make a lot of transformational decisions. But what was the first attempt she made? The first and most important step she took was becoming a student of her biomarkers.

In this chapter of the book, our focus is on discussing the phenomenon of biomarker optimization and getting you acquainted with the eight most essential biomarkers that you need to watch as an AFib patient(s). It also reveals how to optimize every one of them to maximize your chances of putting atrial fibrillation into remission or stop it before it renders you hopeless and perplexed like Stella.

For better understanding, it will be necessary to tell you how it all started. The first and most thorough attempt to describe an integral aspect of science was in a publication: Biological Markers in Epidemiology, put up by the Oxford University Press in 1990. The editors explained how researchers and experts had identified mediums to see an infection long before it was conventionally diagnosable and to monitor its development with simple tests instead of invasive procedures. But then, they issued a warning to prevent people from getting too excited about the paradigm-shifting potential, "considerable groundwork is required to relate biomarkers in tissues readily available for human monitoring".

But there have been significant developments since then. Today, scientists and researchers have seen more than a thousand biomarkers. While the concept 'biomarker' is often described as a chemical and protein in the body that can be measured from the blood, it can also be compared to any health indicator that can be measured over some time to track biological processes. For example, these markers/indicators can be clues to the status, presence, or level of infection. They can also indicate the extent to which a therapy or treatment is working.

So, for an individual whose focus is putting atrial fibrillation into remission, biomarker monitoring is not just important; it's indispensable. That's because a lot of medical problems aren't as binary as a lot many people think. For example, just between good health and suffering AFib are thousands upon millions of small steps that are not discernable by patients or by the conventional methods physicians use to test this condition. However, these steps can now be monitored and followed with the help of biomarkers. So what biomarkers do, is that they help you prioritize what lifestyle optimization methods you should use, determine if ablation is necessary and when to pursue it, and know which medications should be taken and which to avoid.

You've likely had one or more of your biomarkers checked a few times without actually realizing it. For example, prostate-specific antigen, referred to as PSA, is one of the most popularly known biomarkers. PSA is often used to assess and monitor the status of people having or at risk of having prostate cancer. Thus, each time you place your hand in a blood pressure monitor or have the temperature of your body taken or blood is taken from your body for a cholesterol check; you've undergone the process of evaluating your biomarkers to assess your health.

Today, you have an endless range of options guiding biomarker testing. The world market for diagnostic tools and devices that measure biomarkers is available in the tens of millions of dollars and increasing rapidly. As a result, you may spend a while trying to get a test for all your markers. However, whenever atrial fibrillation is concerned, there are just eight necessary blood tests that any physician can order (and some you can choose to do yourself at home). Therefore, it would be best if you get at least one on a semi-regular basis.

You do not need to get all of these biomarkers checked regularly. However, it is safer to get each carried out at the required time and continue to watch out for the ones that are primarily associated with AFib symptoms that you are having. As far as decisions concerning biomarkers are concerned, you can help your doctor a lot if you are knowledgeable about what these diagnoses are, what they mean, and the methods of measuring them.

Anemia Including the Size of the Red Blood Cells

For many years, still uncountable though, anaemia (a medical condition characterized by the lack of red blood cells in the body) has been known to be a severe contributive factor to atrial fibrillation- and can serve as evidence of a more devastating condition. As a result, doctors often test for this biomarker in many of their AFib patients. The problem is that most people don't undergo this test as often as they should to make sure that they are enhancing all of the most vital markers.

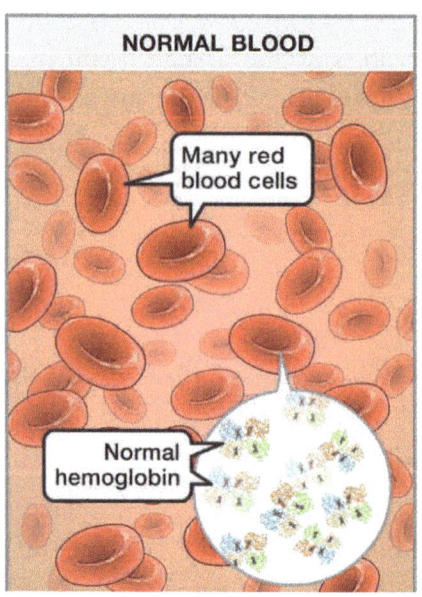
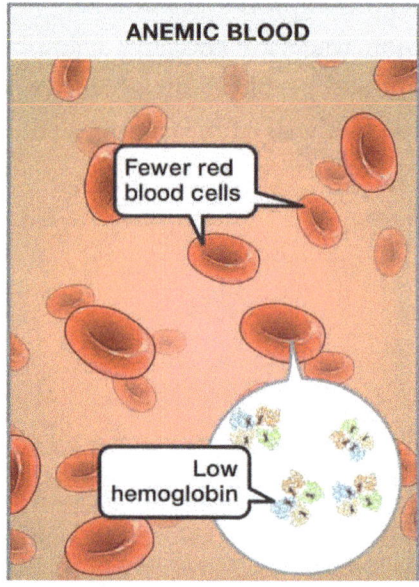

Anaemia is always an outcome of either of two things. First, whether you are losing blood in one area of your body or your bone marrow is incapable of making sufficient red blood cells. In the two cases, the consequence is that your heart is deprived of adequate oxygen and that stress, just like most stress on the heart, increases the risk of AFib.

Although this condition is rarely expected, yet that doesn't mean it should be treated with little or no attention, especially if you have had or at risk of having atrial fibrillation. Even you are an AFib patient on an anticoagulant, which can induce anaemia without any traceable symptoms of blood loss. Not only does anaemia make you more susceptible to having AFib, but it also increases the risk of suffering from other health conditions like a stroke or a heart attack. That is the reason you should be working alongside your doctor to treat the substrate causes of anaemia and reduce the chances of any other bad thing happening if you have been diagnosed with both AFib and anaemia.

The amount of haemoglobin is measured in grams per deciliter (g/dl) of blood through an anaemia test. If you are a man, the normal range is between 13.5 and 17.5 g/dl. Among women, it falls between 12 to 15.5 g/dl. Therefore, you should aim at being in the middle of these ranges at all costs. In addition to these figures, it is also essential that you know the type of anaemia you are suffering from. The type of anaemia depends on the characteristics and size of the red blood cells. For instance, a shortage or decline in the quantity of folate or vitamin B12 can result in a type of anaemia referred to as macrocytic, which means that the few red blood cells carrying oxygen in your body are tremendous. On the other hand, other medical conditions such as deficiency of iron and blood loss can cause microcytic anaemia, which means that the few red blood cells carrying oxygen in your body are microscopic. These types of anaemia can trigger AFib episodes, but as studies have revealed, the treatments for each varies from the other.

You can correct macrocytic anaemia by making life-changing food decisions. All you have to do is increase your intake of vegetables and fish. You can make use of supplements as the case may be. It is also imperative for you to avoid taking medications such as the frequently prescribed proton-pump inhibitors for reflux of acid, which may be hindering the absorption of significant nutrients.

Since microcytic anaemia is often a result of iron deficiency, it is recommended that you feed on more rich foods in iron. These foods help the body in the absorption of iron. Examples of these foods include tofu, spinach, broccoli, dark chocolate, and organic or wild meat. Foods that are not necessarily rich in iron can also be eaten. Examples of such foods are fruits with several vitamins Vs.

Excess red blood cells in the body can affect regular sinus rhythm. It mainly occurs when the body tries as much as possible to live up to lung problems and genetic irregularity such as hemochromatosis by making excess red blood cells. Though this is not common, yet is it worth something to take note of when you are assessing your biomarkers.

Vitamin D

Do you want to feel a little more attached to the universe? You sure are eager to feel some sense of connection, aren't you? Every living thing around you, the building blocks of life existing on the planet, the atomic components mostly found inside you- the carbon, oxygen, hydrogen, sulfur, nitrogen, and phosphorus are also elements available in their large numbers in our galaxy. The Milky Way galaxy and Homo sapiens are said to have a lot in common, so much that they are composed of nearly 97 per cent of similar kinds of atoms. This is according to the facts revealed by astronomers who listed more than 140,000 stars for the Sloan Digital Sky Survey. Hence, we are cosmic dust.

So, it is pretty interesting to know that one of the best things we can do to maintain stable and good health is getting outside and soak up some sunshine. Is it hard to believe that failure to obtain sufficient vitamin D (a hormone created in the body when ultraviolet rays of the sun penetrate the skin) in quantity required by the body can put your health in danger? A low vitamin D level is said to put you at risk of suffering many chronic health conditions, and AFib is not left out of the list. Studies have revealed that a deficiency in Vitamin D can increase the susceptibility to atrial fibrillation by 31 per cent. This perhaps is due to heightened inflammation via vitamin D receptors on fluid balance, cardiac cells, and altered calcium reaction. If you are already prone to having AFib, that shouldn't be seen as a mere consideration.

Fortunately, among the many biomarkers to optimize, vitamin D happens to be the easiest to treat and correct for most patients. For people who, due to one reason or the other, might not be able to get enough sunshine or those who don't eat many dairy products, mushrooms, and fish, supplements can be a good option. However, nothing as promising as taking a long walk under the sun's smiling face. Just taking twelve to fifteen minutes to walk under the sun can work a lot of magic on the level of your vitamin D. It gives you exposure to the sun, although it must be moderate depending on your doctor's instruction. Doctors will determine, among others, the distance from the equator, the period or season of the year, and whether you live at a higher elevation or sea level.

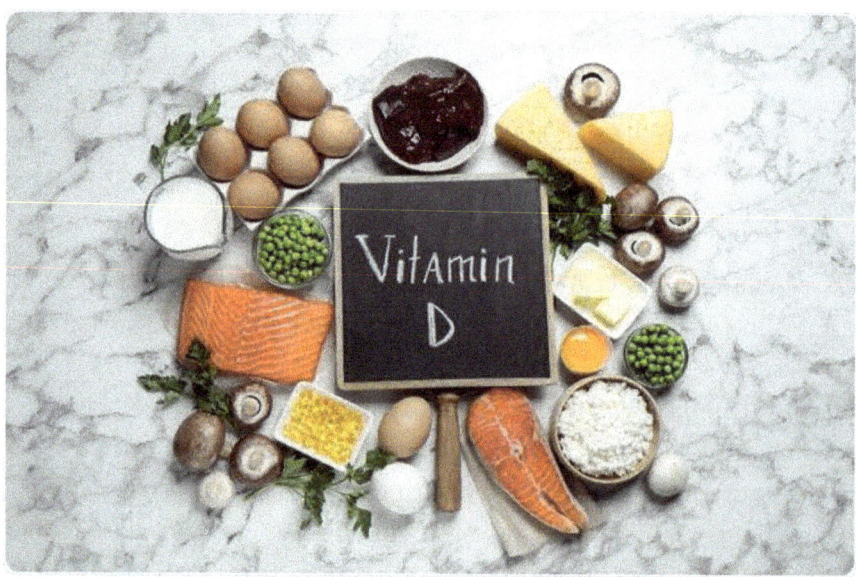

The question now is, "how high does your level of Vitamin D need to be?". While there is some argument about whether a target of 20 to 30 nanograms per deciliter (ng/dl) is okay, anything less than 20 ng/dl is certainly too small. The assertion by naturopaths and most integrative doctors of 50- to 70- ng/dl range is also good.

So, why do you need the diagnosis? Why not take a vitamin D supplement every day instead of taking a walk under the sun? It is because taking a walk under the sun comes with a lot of natural benefits. Even research has shown that taking a vitamin D supplement (anything above 100 ng/dl) may increase your risk of having atrial fibrillation by a two and a half chance.

C-Reactive Protein

A research carried out on more than 2000 people and published in 2009 indicated that a type of biomarker referred to as C-reactive protein or CRP for short was a potential predictor of who would have AFib. To many people, the outcome of this research was surprising. The reason for this surprise was because CRP has little or no connection with the heart. Instead, it is mainly produced in the liver, and it's usually used as a blood test indicator for inflammation.

The relationship between inflammation and a condition commonly linked to the heart's irregular triggering of electrical impulses is yet to be established. But, it turned out to be something worth looking into. While the primary mechanistic associations are yet to be fully understood, experts believe that AFib could be both a cause and an outcome of inflammation. It is a very terrible example of a "lethal cycle" in which scarring of the heart causes inflammation (severally because of the movement of immune cells against bruised tissues) and may result in severe heart scarring.

CRP can be a significantly helpful biomarker as a result of this association. Yet, of all the tests that physicians can recommend for AFib, CRP is likely the most frequently overlooked. Unlike other tests, CRP is relatively cheaper and can disclose the overall risks linked to AFib.

If you have ever had this test carried out on you, you might be aware that there are just two types of it. The first type is the standard CRP, which is most suitable for finding inflammation linked to autoimmune infections. The second type is the highly sensitive CRP (hs-CRP), which is ideal for finding inflammation of the heart. The results of these diagnoses do not always contradict each other; they match so well. For example, if the CRP is relatively high, the hs-CRP will likely be increased also. In the same vein, a low CRP will result in a low hs-CRP. The fact that they produce similar outcomes does not mean that you can switch one for the other to track the rate of your progress. For instance, a CRP test is done in February, and a hs-CRP test carried out in August will likely be counterproductive; you won't see any tangible outcome. However, if your doctor chooses to do one and do the other at a later date, for any reason best known to him, you are still in safe hands.

The unit of measurements for both tests is milligrams per litre (mg/L). Doctors who treat atrial fibrillation patients and recognize the value of this biomarker always come across some very high CRPs (anything higher than three mg/L), while a healthy CRP is almost unable to be detected. The stable number here is 1. If your CRP is way above one mg/L, you will have to work on ways to reduce your risks. You do not need to be afraid if suddenly your CRP goes high. It will go back to normal all by itself. It's just trying to let you know that an "inflammation fire" is burning in one part of your body, and the immune system is working to put the situation under control. Although such an occurrence could have resulted from AFib, several other factors could be responsible, including an untested autoimmune disease, a viral infection, bad genetics, a tedious exercise, and cancer. More often than not, eating and lifestyle choices have resulted in severe unhealthy activation of the immune system and compounded AFib.

If you are interested in reducing your CRP to the lowest possible ebb, there's just a single thing you need to do: cut some inches off your waist. Waist size monitors very closely to visceral fat, including all kinds of fats stored in the torso- also in the pericardium, a membranous and thin sac that holds the heart. The pericardial fat layer encompassing the heart can be very thick, even an inch thick.

What this fat does is that it releases cytokines which are responsible for inducing inflammation. Everyone has a different body size, and for that reason, research has shown that to reduce the risk of visceral fat, men should get their waist size to less than thirty-five inches. In comparison, women, on the other should target below thirty-two inches.

Cutting some inches off your waist isn't the only ideal way of controlling a high CRP. Other tracks such as daily exercise, taking an anti-inflammatory diet, getting enough sleep, avoiding stress at all costs will also help you to reduce your CRP and keep it at your desired stake.

Thyroid Panel

You know George Herbert Walker Bush, the forty-first president of the United States who lived a healthy and happy life in his nineties. Even until the end, he was always in good health. Yet, at an age when a large number of people would have had their feet in the ground, the onetime president still had his head in the clouds. So what could be more satisfying than celebrating your eightieth and ninetieth birthday skydiving?

However, the reverse was the case when he was in his mid-sixties. He was the president and had several incidents of health woes due to his age. He was diagnosed with AFib while he was still in the White House.

What can you deduce from here? First, being a president can be a whole lot of stress. A brief look at the before-and-after images of US presidents will show you something astounding. And it is no new news that psychological stress is a significant factor that induces atrial fibrillation. Yet Bush's atrial fibrillation could not have been said to have been triggered by stress alone; instead, it was firstly a result of a hyperactive thyroid.

Hyperthyroidism happens when the thyroid gland, a ductless gland located in the neck region secrets hormones necessary for the body cells' proper functioning, begins to produce the thyroid hormone in excess. Under normal circumstances, this hormone aids metabolism (something good), but when it is overactive, or you have been prescribed too much of it, it becomes a potent stimulant. As time passes by, its outcome often includes anxiety, tremors, weight loss, and several other serious issues. Also, it can lead to palpitations and abnormal heartbeats. Sound familiar? Yes, hyperthyroidism and AFib are closely related. Not only does thyroid hormone induce atrial fibrillation, but it also alters the chemistry of your blood in such a way that your body quickly produces blood clots, thereby making hyperthyroidism and AFib a double whammy that results in stroke.

An underactive thyroid can also trigger AFib. To make things worse, just a superficial irregularity in any of your thyroid hormones can subject you to the risk of atrial fibrillation even if you were once in good health and without symptoms. That's the bad news.

The good news is that once an irregularity in the thyroid hormone has been diagnosed, it can easily be corrected. In this regard, the first thing to do is knowing your thyroid panel. It often includes a diagnosis for thyroid-inciting hormones like thyroxine and triiodothyronine (referred to as TSH, free T4, and free T3, respectively). Your goal is to work to ensure your numbers are all within the normal ranges.

Just like other biomarkers, you can always choose to make more advanced thyroid diagnoses. However, if you intend to make the diagnosis through your doctor, then a deep knowledge about the levels of your TSH, T3, and T4 are always enough to provide you with the data you need to reduce your stroke and AFib risks. You may do these tests at home as well. You might have some cash to dash out.

Moreover, because hyperthyroidism can be a sign of AFib, it's not out of place to find a newly tested AFib patient to have been prescribed a thyroid hormone. If you belong to this category, you need to do your thyroid panel again. It is because research has shown that high doses of thyroid hormones can increase the risks of AFib. Another problem often treated that can lead to more atrial fibrillation and thyroid irregularities is iodine deficiency. Although this problem was once only evident in developing nations, it is gradually resurfacing in more economically developed countries.

The reason is not far-fetched: there is no iodization of most of the salt used in processed foods. Thus, if you do not want seaweed, seafood, strawberries, dairy, or iodized salt is not used in your home salt shaker, or you are not used to taking multivitamins containing iodine risk is very high.

Hemoglobin A1C

A lot of people appear to know that high blood sugar can spell doom for those with diabetes. What isn't clear to them is that glucose, the raw sugar that acts as one of their bodies' most frequent energy sources, is an essential biomarker for several other medical conditions, including AFib. People with diabetes are 50 per cent more vulnerable to atrial fibrillation. In addition, the longer you have diabetes, or the higher the blood glucose continues to rise, the more likely you are to have AFib. The problem is that long before you are diagnosed with diabetes, high blood sugar might have tampered with the heart's electrical system.

Hemoglobin A1c

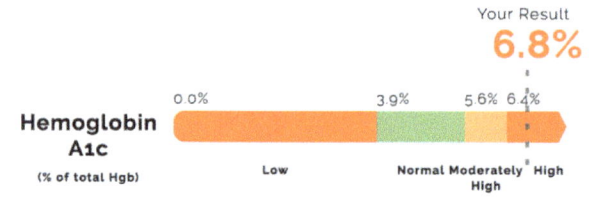

Your Result
6.8%

Hemoglobin A1c
(% of total Hgb)

0.0% 3.9% 5.6% 6.4%

Low Normal Moderately High
High

When your result falls within the high range, it may be a sign of pre-diabetes and you should discuss the status of your sugar metabolism with your doctor. If you have already been told that you have diabetes this is consistent with controlled diabetes. Always seek the advice of your doctor or qualified healthcare provider if you have any questions about your result.

The underlying causes of this relationship are yet to be precise. However, some researchers and experts suggested that it is not the level of the blood glucose but the fluctuation of those levels that increases the formation of a gene known as TXNIP. This gene, as a result, causes an increase in the ranks of reactive molecules that can trigger the death of cells- a developmental response, perhaps to the needs of the body to prevent the growth and spread of dangerous microbes. Thus, like a thinking process, the body treats the waning and waxing of glucose like an invasion, bringing out all the steps- including the death of some healthy cells- to fight it. The consequence attached to the end of a heart cell is fibrosis, which may hinder the heart's normal and smooth electrical conduction.

Fibrosis isn't the only bad outcome of a high glucose level. Insulin resistance and glucose intolerance have been revealed to be responsible for abnormal thickening and enlargement of the heart. And just like diabetes can damage the nerves and tissues in the feet and hands, it can also destroy the nerves and tissues in the heart, leading to AFib.

Having a simple understanding of these relationships is essential for the process of taking ownership of the therapies and treatments used to move these biomarkers in healthier directions. Still, it's necessary to recall that this can happen in whatever way possible. Therefore, it is indispensable for patients or people at risk of having atrial fibrillation to get tested regularly for haemoglobin A1C. Haemoglobin measures the quantity of glucose in the body sticking to the red blood cells over a couple of months, valued as a percentage.

Sugarcoating foods such as chocolate doughnuts and gumdrops is good, but it's not safe for the red blood cells. Thus, the inference is clear: the lower the average A1C percentage, the safer. Also, studies have tried to establish a connection between A1C and the risk of having an AFib stroke.

An A1C reading above 5.7 per cent is said to be prediabetes, and above 6.5 shows diabetes. Therefore, to reduce the risk of having AFib, you should strive for an A1C below 5.7. In addition, many people have realized that any processed carbohydrate, such as those found in flour, is easily digested by the body to form sugar, and this process of digestion process takes just a few minutes. Therefore, even wheat bread, which is termed "healthy" can spike your blood glucose levels.

Eating late at night can also be very unfavorable to the levels of your A1C. Unlike a body in motion, a body at rest can't process and convert sugar effectively. And that's a clue that is moving from one place to another is an essential factor for keeping the level of sugar at a relatively low ebb. So when do you usually take your last meal of the day? Usually, it should come at least three hours before the time you head to your bedroom, and it is inevitably essential to spend few hours out of that in-between time doing some physical activities. There are just too many fun ways to go about that.

Whichever eating pattern or diet you choose to fight against your A1C levels, you shouldn't do away with some doses of exercise, which are vital in lowering your weight to normal levels.

Comprehensive Metabolic Panel

You should know by now that AFib isn't heart disease. Instead, it is an abnormality or infection of the body that distinctively affects the heart. Having learned that, do you think a test that gives a comprehensive overview of the numerous functions of the body is needed? Of course, yes. This is the reason if you have AFib or you have been diagnosed with it, your physician or his regular counterpart who treated your atrial fibrillation attack has perhaps already recommended a comprehensive metabolic panel or put CMP.

Many people do this battery of blood tests as an integral part of their yearly physical. Unfortunately, however, most Americans don't get physicals year after year, and many doctors believe that these annual activities are counterproductive and even unnecessary ways of taking care of one's health. And even AFib patients usually go longer between physician visits than they ought to. But with the aid of a comprehensive metabolic panel, you will be able to have enough information on various biomarkers.

Although this test varies from one lab to another, it is one sure way of measuring the levels of your blood sugar and electrolytes, as well as the functions of your liver and kidneys. Since the importance of knowing your blood sugar levels has been considered in the previous paragraphs, let's focus on other areas.

Electrolytes

These include all elements and chemicals such as potassium, sodium, magnesium, chloride, and calcium, which are helpful in the conduction of electrical impulses in the body. If you should ponder upon the roles performed by these elements, you will know how vital they are in addressing AFib. Since the depletion of electrolytes is one of the underlying factors that cause atrial fibrillation, electrolyte optimization is critical in maintaining a regular sinus rhythm. The reason electrolytes are so helpful in keeping the heart in rhythm is because the electrical channels in each cell of the heart depend on the average balance of electrolytes to work actively.

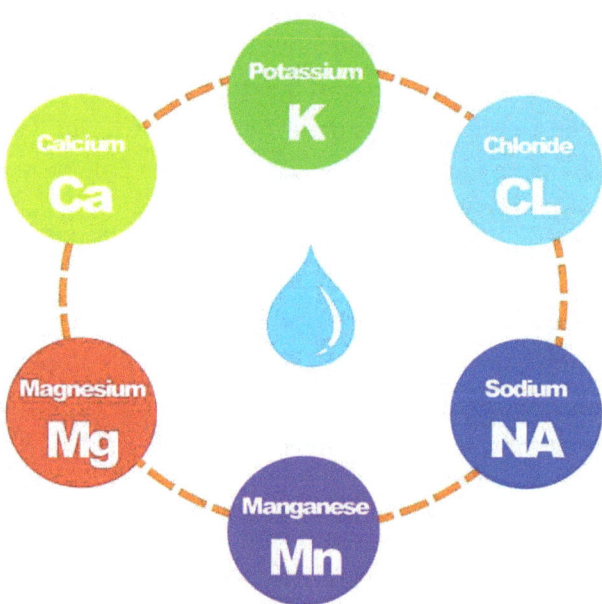

What's the level of your electrolytes? Are you high or low? Well, when it comes to AFib, a low level of electrolytes may not be good. But it is often easy to correct.

As far as preventing atrial fibrillation is concerned, there are just two electrolytes that play a vital role. The first is potassium, and the second is magnesium. Not only do these electrolytes play a critical role in the prevention of AFib, but they are also helpful in keeping track of your antiarrhythmic medications prescription.

Concerning potassium, you have to keep the levels close to four millimoles per liter (mmol/L). As studies and research have indicated, this level affords the heart to function well. For magnesium, the class should not be less than 2 milligrams per deciliter (mg/dL). Having the level of your serum magnesium stay above this value can significantly reduce your chances of developing atrial fibrillation by as much as 50 percent. They can also help with many other biomarkers, including blood pressure and CRP. Magnesium can be pretty unpredictable, though. After all, more significant parts are found in the cells because a tiny amount is contained in the bloodstream. It is why blood diagnosis misses up to ninety-nine (99) percent of the amount of magnesium in your body.

So, why do we see people with relatively low levels of electrolytes? There are two most common reasons. Firstly, they are used to eating electrolyte-depleted food. Secondly, they are used to taking diuretics (a medication used for blood retention against heart failure, high blood pressure, and other causes). You don't have to rob Paul to pay Peter when it comes to taking diuretic medications because strict adherence to the approaches and procedures for beating AFib analyzed in this book may completely abrogate your need to take diuretics. You will be doing yourself a lot good by simply eating foods that are rich in electrolytes. Foods ranging from avocados to bananas and from butternut squash to spinach can help in this regard. Magnesium and potassium supplements can be needed in some cases.

"What about sport drinks like Powerade and Gatorade? Aren't they helpful?". I've been asked this question several times by different people. Although these sports drinks contain a large number of electrolytes and can relatively raise the level of electrolytes in your body, they can also increase your blood sugar status. Even soft drinks (which are artificially sweetened) have more risks attached than benefits. But if the rate of your potassium is relatively low, let's say from 3.5 to 3.9 mmol/L, you can correct the deficiency by simply increasing your intake of vegetables and fruits. As long as your kidneys are in good shape, it is almost impossible to have excess potassium by eating healthy foods.

Deficiency in Liver and Kidney Functions

This is one of the factors that has been alluded to cause AFib, although research is yet to establish if liver and kidney problems are potential causes of atrial fibrillation, or if AFib can be responsible for kidney and liver deficit, or it's simply another vicious cycle. Irrespective of the situation, the fact remains that poor liver and kidney functions can raise your risk. Thus, if the goal is to beat atrial fibrillation at its game, and enjoy the bliss of good health afterwards, then you have to optimize both liver and kidney functions. In this regard, the CMP can be pretty invaluable.

Having your liver and kidney function in good shape can also reduce the risk of any drug you are taking or have been prescribed by your doctor. For instance, poor liver and kidney functions may increase both chances of bleeding and the odds of life-threatening ventricular arrhythmia; perhaps you have been prescribed an antiarrhythmic. If either of these organs isn't working as expected, you should see a hepatologist for your liver or a nephrologist for your kidneys. If you live in a remote area, a trip to a nearby city to see an expert can save you the risk.

Homocysteine

You are perhaps aware that protein is one of the basic building blocks of life and that without amino acids, the body can't make or produce protein. You are probably also aware that an excess amount of amino acids in your body system can signify that you are suffering from a condition known as "omnivore's dilemma" because the meat is mainly available globally. There's no enough time to consume it. Of course, all of this means that it's vital to know the level of your amino acids, yet, a straightforward blood test for one of the most dangerous amino acids, Homocysteine, is seldom done.

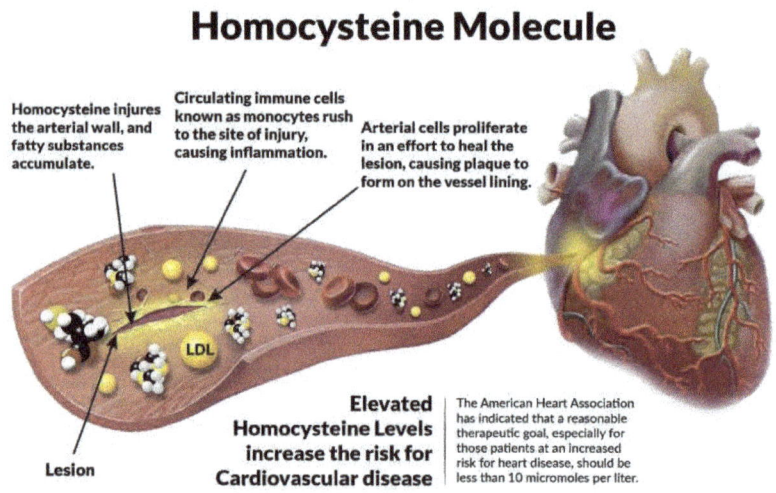

Homocysteine Molecule

Homocysteine injures the arterial wall, and fatty substances accumulate.

Circulating immune cells known as monocytes rush to the site of injury, causing inflammation.

Arterial cells proliferate in an effort to heal the lesion, causing plaque to form on the vessel lining.

LDL

Lesion

Elevated Homocysteine Levels increase the risk for Cardiovascular disease

The American Heart Association has indicated that a reasonable therapeutic goal, especially for those patients at an increased risk for heart disease, should be less than 10 micromoles per liter.

Like every other biomarker discussed, the exact mechanism that guarantees that this amino can induce AFib has not been established. Still, studies have suggested that too much of this amino acid can be destructive to collagen, which provides elasticity and structure to the heart. This is a vital feature of a muscle that's always in motion, and the outcome of this can be atrial enlargement and cardiac scarring. Research has also shown that this dangerous amino: Homocysteine has the risk of killing cells that decorate the inside of the heart and arteries. That's too bad because an excessive amount of Homocysteine in the blood has been linked with dementia, heart attack, stroke, and- no surprise this time- atrial fibrillation.

A healthy level of Homocysteine should be measured at ten micromoles per litre (umol/L). Anything more than that should make you eager to seek correction.

Reducing the level of this biomarker isn't a difficult task. So long as you are still getting adequate vitamin B12- which is found in animal protein, you also have to reduce the number of land animals you consume. Other healthy things that can help include vitamin B12 from spinach, sweet potatoes, banana, sunflower seeds, and folate derived from beans and green leafy vegetables. Some individuals also think there's a more straightforward way of going about this, including taking B6, B12, and folic acid supplements. While you may think that taking vitamin supplements can reduce the amount of Homocysteine, tests conducted on two patients who had had heart failure suggest that these supplements have little or no benefit.

Highly Sensitive Troponin

The last test that can be a valuable biomarker for people with atrial fibrillation or those who are at risk of developing it is highly sensitive troponin or hs-TN for short. If you have ever been taken to the emergency room during an AFib attack, then you've likely taken this test already. Generally, the average level of troponin should not be more than 0.4 ng/mL.

Since troponin is a heart muscle protein that signifies tremendous damage in the heart muscles, and increased troponin rate in the bloodstream is a negative sign, a terrible sign. A high amount of troponin in a person with AFib can increase the risk of heart failure, heart attack, stroke, or untimely death. This is why it is crucial for anyone with a high amount of troponin to be closely watched. This can't be overemphasized- a high amount of troponin is a great disaster. Thus, it might be tough for you to put your atrial fibrillation into remission if you have an increased troponin level.

Is all hope lost? Not at all. With aggressive and prompt therapy and lifestyle optimization, the level of troponin can reduce relatively.

Chapter Two

Confronting AFIB: Living a Better Life

Recall back in part one when you evaluated the different substrate factors that put people at high risk of developing atrial fibrillation? There is a lot of work to be done for those causes. If you are finding it difficult to get enough sleep, for example, you will like to give due attention to the section that focuses on rest, or if you are too engaged such that you are often stressed, the area on stress is all for you.

But, you'll also do well to remember that AFib doesn't come from just a single source. A struggle in one section of your health may worsen an initially milder effort, and the human body, just like a machine, is more challenging to get back into working track once something has gone wrong. Thus, if you have been diagnosed with atrial fibrillation, all the steps and procedures in this chapter are particularly indispensable.

That means exposing you to the various factors preventing you from having restorative and healthy sleep, finding ways to reduce adverse stress, taking the critical steps you need to reduce weight, and putting an end to unhealthy habits such as smoking. In this chapter, the strategies for bringing all of these goals to reality are expounded.

You can take a step-by-step approach. You don't need to follow the order provided here. Since you know the causes of your arrhythmia, adopt the sequence that suits you. But if, in the long run, your goal is to put your AFib into remission and prevent it from resurfacing, you may need to put all the approaches into effect. And while an optimized lifestyle may not be sufficient to put your atrial fibrillation into remission, it can make ablation or antiarrhythmic medications far more effective than they would have been.

That's the goal of lifestyle optimization: not only to address each of these parts of your life but doing so in such a way that guarantees that your health and life improve and get better over time. What's more important than this? Recall that failure to address your AFib will make your condition get worse and worse over time.

Also, you have to know that lifestyle optimization isn't a thing you do one time and refuse to come back to; you have to do it over and over again, probably until the time it becomes a habit- at that point, you can't do without it anymore. The things you are able and willing to do to improve your health will set you up for success later in the future.

So, what do you do to confront your atrial fibrillation?

Get Enough Sleep

Initially, Debbie wasn't willing to tell her doctor what the causes of her AFib were.

You can recall from part one that she couldn't grasp why an assessment of the underlying factors responsible for her AFib was so necessary. Immediately she learned why it was required; it didn't take long for her to discover two underlying factors: weight and sleep.

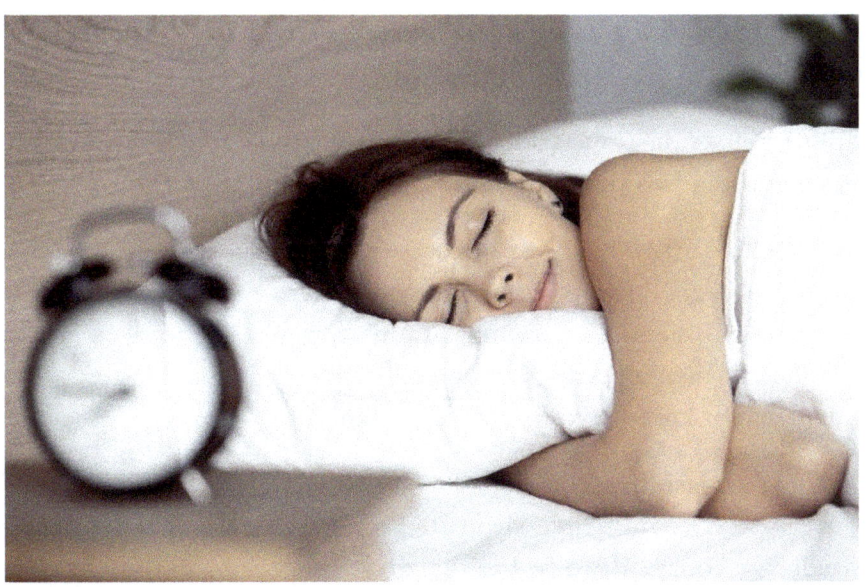

She knew that if she fought and won the battle against atrial fibrillation, she would have to take some bold steps in addressing these two factors. She had been taking steps to reduce her weight, and that wasn't a problem. She also had the view that sleep was going to be an easy thing to deal with. Then, it became apparent to her that sleep could be an integral factor in reducing her weight. Studies have revealed that better and enough sleep can lead to a massive reduction of up to 520 calories from an individual's daily food intake, unlike their sleep-deprived counterparts. Significantly sleep-deprived people do not only eat more food; they also often eat late at night, and eating late at night can be pretty unhealthy and cause weight gain.

"Before then, I hadn't even thought about the essential role sleep played in this regard," she remembered. "So, I immediately understood the whole thing and learned about the studies that reveal such a strong association between AFib and the quality of sleep I was having, it didn't take me long to realize that I wasn't having enough sleep."

"But I was wrong," she said. "Having better and enough sleep was more complicated than I thought. You have to work for it".

Yes, Debbie might have been wrong about how easy it was to have sufficient sleep, but she wasn't wrong about how vital it was to make time to sleep. The amount of time you set aside to sleep is significant when it comes to your general wellbeing, and more uniquely, for keeping your heart in rhythm.

This is the reason sleep was made the first factor to be considered in this chapter. Because unless you are having enough and better sleep needed by your body to be healthy, every other thing in this chapter will be pretty challenging to achieve. The amount of sleep varies from person to person, but there's almost no person on earth who cannot benefit from having at least seven hours of sleep per night. And to be specific, that's seven hours of better sleep, absolutely free of sleep disruptions- not just being in bed for seven good hours.

Therefore, you need to plan your sleep. So, how do you go about that?

- **Schedule your sleep**

You should take a look at your calendar. Suppose, like most individuals, you have blocks of time reserved for vacations. In that case, work, dinner with family and friends, visits from friends and other relatives, as well as a whole lot of different things, do you at all have a block of seven hours dedicated explicitly to sleeping to reduce your risk of having AFib?

For many people, rather than having a block of time, they imply some hours for sleep. If lack of sufficient and regular sleep is one of the underlying factors for your AFib, you need to join the ten percent of Americans who make their sleep a top priority. Studies have revealed that just a night of poor sleep can heighten your risk of an AFib episode the next day by threefold. And the best way to ensure that you have a sufficient sleep is by making use of your calendar.

Just as you do everything in your capacity to ensure that you aren't late to work, you should also do everything to ensure that you don't go to bed late. Although simple, yet it is the most robust approach to take. Research has also shown that the simple act of setting a bedtime and adhering to it results in an additional hour of sleep every night.

Do not forget the target: seven hours of sleep per night, not for the time in bed. If it takes you a relatively long time to fall asleep, let's say about 30 minutes, and you also have a midnight awakening to check if the doors were actually locked, or use the restroom, or drink some water, or for whatever reason, you should perhaps fix eight hours per night.

- **Lights Out**

Having a block of time reserved for sleep isn't enough; there are other things you have to make sure are in order. For instance, if you are a police officer, showing up at your duty post isn't enough; you have to make sure that your uniform, your badge, your body camera, amongst other accessories of the work, are all in place. Sleep is the same thing.

Setting up a bedtime is vital, but once you are in bed, you must ensure that everything is in place to do what you ought to be doing there. It involves maintaining a calm, quiet, and clean room with a lot of fresh air. It also includes having in mind the purpose of going to bed: sleep. If there's something else, you should do it elsewhere.

To be very straight on this subject: your bed isn't a place to have your meal. It isn't the right place to do your work/job, and it isn't also the right place for any "screentime." While exposure to any light can diminish the making of melatonin: a hormone that assists the body to control its sleep-wake cycle, blue light (the part of the spectrum frequently emitted by computer and television screens) can exacerbate it. Hence, the presence of an electronic device in your bedroom can rob you of an hour of sleep each night. Contrarily, by simply removing the television or computer from your bedroom and committing yourself to not taking a mobile phone or any other device into that sacred room, you can reset the watch, so to say, from seven hours to eight hours of sleep per night.

- **Regulate the Chemicals**

Everyone's quite aware that some chemicals can hinder quality of sleep. The majority of these chemicals are found in energy drinks we consume. Take, for instance, caffeine. Caffeine can affect your sleep badly, but still, many people do not think about these effects. More than you view it; caffeine isn't just a stimulant; it is a potent substance that can last for as long as a day in your body's system. For some people, the significant parts of the effects that come with it are unnoticed within five hours. Still, about 50 percent of people possess a variant of a gene called CYPIA2, which reduces the quantity of a specific enzyme of the liver to a point where the body metabolizes caffeine gradually. For many people who prioritize their bedtime, a "caffeine restriction," which is observed six hours before bedtime, is a good principle. However, the best way to ensure that caffeine doesn't affect your sleep is to avoid taking it at all.

Alcohol is another chemical or substance that can disrupt your sleep. If this doesn't make any sense to you yet, wait for it. Unlike the effects that come with caffeine, alcohol is a depressant of the central nervous system. And yes, the claim that a drink before going to bed makes some people fall asleep quickly is valid, but that benefit is induced by reducing the amount of sleep they have. Research has shown that people who drink alcohol before going to bed have less REM sleep: rest, which includes dreaming, rapid eye movement, and bodily action. This type of sleep offers the most significant benefits in terms of restfulness and general health. REM is also essential in keeping the heart in rhythm. For example, a study has shown that people who get less REM sleep are more vulnerable to AFib, with the chances of increasing as REM level decreases.

- **Address Sleep Apnea**

Although you may have blocks of time set aside for sleep and ensure all lights or screens are out; still, you will find yourself struggling with quality sleep. It is a condition called sleep apnea and does not matter if you reduce your intake of caffeine, alcohol, and other chemical substances.

Discovering that you have sleep apnea may be pretty tricky, because more often than not, the symptoms of this sleep disorder are not easily noticeable. And perhaps these symptoms are apparent; many people still can't decipher that they are related to sleep apnea. Individuals suffering from sleep apnea usually snore like a bear, breathless, and then struggle for air. In some categories of people, sleep apnea symptoms can be very subtle, in which case the center of their brain is dysfunctional. For individuals suffering from this type of sleep apnea, their sleep is often restful, deep, and seemingly quiet. Unless you are paying close attention to them while sleeping, you hardly notice them struggling for breath. In all types of sleep apnea, these times of breathlessness cause blood oxygen levels to drop, thereby increasing the risk of coronary artery disease, high blood pressure, heart failure, and atrial fibrillation.

If you are yet to be convinced that you are suffering from sleep apnea, you should consider answering these five questions in all sincerity: do you snore? Do you experience extreme tiredness during the day and want to take a nap? Do you have excess weight? Have you been diagnosed with high blood pressure? Do you have a big neck of about 16 inches or 17 inches in circumference for women and men, respectively? If you answered "yes" to the five questions, you are at risk of sleep apnea. If you answered "yes" to three out of the five questions, you are also at risk and should pay a visit to your doctor to help you in this regard.

- **Have a Warm Bath**

More often than not, people resort to taking alcohol to get rid of stress and relax. They are not aware that there are several other healthy means of going about relaxation that can even benefit the quality of their sleep. Taking a warm shower or bath at a temperature of 104° can improve the time it takes you to start sleeping, the quality of your sleep, and how long your sleep lasts, as well as how often you wake up in the night.

Are you the type of person who needs a shower in the morning to have a good day? That's a good habit, and you should keep it up. Cultivate taking a warm evening bath as well. That will make your sleep better and sound.

Reduce Your Weight

There's no cause of AFib that is common to every person on earth. However, there's a characteristic that is common among all AFib patients: excess weight. Apart from the twenty or thirty-year-olds whose AFib must have been induced by familial factors, and athletes who engage in endurance sports who have been said to suffer AFib due to the nature of their job, it is often rare to see a person at a healthy weight with AFib.

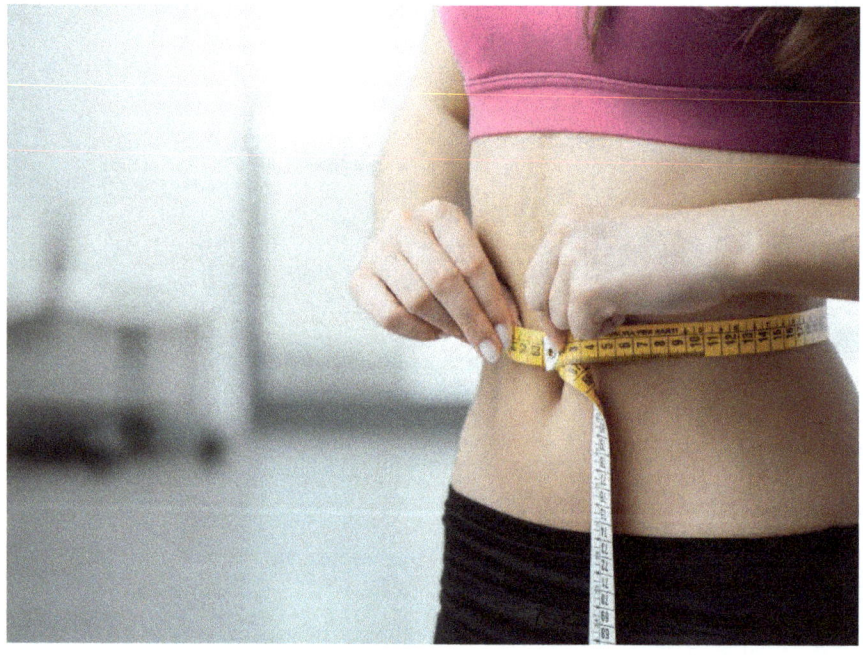

Yet, you can't say that weight itself is the problem. It isn't straightforward. Weight is a strong indicator that shows that the balance between constructive metabolism (this occurs when you eat food) and destructive metabolism (this takes place when the food is digested and used by the body) is probably out of sync. It also indicates that the amount of fat in the body is too much. For example, suppose your heart is surrounded by too much fat. In that case, that can be a big problem because these fats often release harmful cytokines, which makes it more difficult for the muscles at the center of the circulatory system (which seldom gets rest to start with) to perform their job.

Losing weight to many people seems like an impossible goal to accomplish. Although people can reduce their weight by using any diet that controls caloric intake, yet that weight seldom stays off. So, while you might lose some weight this year, you're likely to put up that weight in the coming year. Hence, the diet approach is a temporary one.

Those who are highly overweight, let's say more than one hundred pounds, often resort to weight-loss surgery, popularly referred to as bariatric surgery, to get rid of their weight. There are several ways of going about this, but the most popular is gastric bypass surgery. During this surgery, the small intestine rearrangement and the division of the stomach precede into sections. If that sounds like a complicated thing to do, then it is because many risks and side effects are attached to it. But it can be of great benefit to people fighting AFib or those who do not want it to rear its ugly head. In addition, several kinds of research have shown that bariatric surgery can put atrial fibrillation into remission.

However, you should know that bariatric surgery is a significantly drastic step that can alter your physiology. Before you think of doing that, you should know that there are several other ways you can choose to lose weight without having to change natural features. To optimize this area of your life, a combination of exercise, food, and other lifestyle habits will be of great benefit.

- **Weigh Yourself Daily**

All eight of the blood-based biomarkers discussed in the antecedent chapter are indispensable, and understanding them, as well as monitoring them over time, is crucial to putting AFib into remission. However, if an individual was limited, perhaps because of a reason or another, focusing on only one should be the figure on their bathroom scale. So, yes, weight can be a significant biomarker that should be adequately monitored.

Although the benefits of daily monitoring of body weight are supported by research, there is no need for a scientific study to grasp why this approach works. People who weigh themselves regularly are getting a collection of data and a reminder to ensure that corrective measures are taken when things aren't going in the desired direction. There have been several cases of people who could reduce their weight by simply adopting the principle of checking their weight day after day.

Why does this principle work so well? First, it gives people the opportunity to know what to do concerning their weight. For instance, you can choose to do a little bit more exercise the next day or watch the composition of the food you eat closely. Second, just the simple act of weighing yourself every day almost unintentionally sets off a series of behaviors that ensure that maintaining a healthy body weight becomes much more manageable.

If you are not convenient with stepping on a scale daily to measure your weight, there are several other ways you can go about it. For example, you can employ a fitness coach or get engaged in commercial weight loss programs. Technology has also made things a lot easier; with the aid of an app or notebook available on your smartphone, you can measure your weight. Food journals can also be of great help in this regard.

The amount of bodyweight you need to lose to reduce your risk of atrial fibrillation is not fixed because healthy body weight differs from one person to another. But to be frank, a large number of people with AFib have their weight above the specified body mass index. And while this (BMI) isn't compelling evidence of how healthy a person's body weight is, it is often a good target. So, if you have added more weight in recent years, you will need to lose more than you think you should.

Instead of being discouraged about the amount of weight you need to lose, know that any amount helps. Even losing as little as 3 percent of your body weight daily counts.

- **More Healthy Diets**

Healthy food, uniquely designed for people with AFib, is undoubtedly essential in losing weight and keeping it off over time. However, it would help if you understood that good health doesn't imply low calories. As far as bringing your mechanism into sync is concerned, you need to stop focusing on calories. You should also know that the diet someone else is following, helping such a person lose weight, might not work well with you. But, if you have been used to a particular diet for a long time (meaning you have been watching your weight closely and observing a significant drop), then just like in many cases, there's no reason you should stop doing it. After all, the goal is to eliminate some excess weight that isn't giving your heart enough room to breathe. Across world, people have successfully reduced their weight and kept it off. You have to know what works for you.

Apart from the instance cited above, you can know what works for you from your family members. Again, this is because you guys share some genetic components. If your sibling, for instance, was able to lose weight by eating a particular food, that might work for you, too. Likewise, if your spouse has had a significant reduction in weight by choosing to eat a diet, you should consider taking that as well. After all, partners share a meal, and unlike siblings, they possess more similar gut microbiomes.

Whatever decision you make about your diets, make sure you eat more vegetables, minimize or avoid eating processed and fast foods, sugar, and flour. You will be doing your health and body weight a lot of favor if you do this. And if it turns out to be working for you, and other biomarkers are active as they should, continue and don't stop.

Do More Exercise

Studies have indicated that regular exercise is the number one factor responsible for stable and healthy body weight. However, you should know that exercise alone is not compelling enough as a tool for losing weight. That's because, unlike the belief of many people, the exhausting exercise burns little or no-calorie at all. For example, a race across a mile might burn up to 100 calories. The equivalent of that is a 26.2-mile marathon. And you hardly see people running a marathon- even for the fact that they aren't athletes. The not-so-encouraging news is that even if you choose to run a marathon tomorrow, you are likely not to lose more than a pound of fat. The equation is simple; if you want to lose 20 pounds in the next 20 weeks, you should take part in 20 marathons.

That equation seems rather hard to solve. Yes, it is. Because if at all you choose to get yourself involved in such, your body will need something in return: food. The more exercise you do, the more distance you cover, the hungrier you are likely to get, and the more food you need to eat.

In simpler terms, if you are 180 pounds currently, you are not likely to get down to 175 pounds just by exercising. However, if your healthy food habits lead to weight loss, exercise will prevent the weight from coming back.

Since many people who shed weight tend to gain it back in just a few days, you must be consistent with your feeding and exercise habits. So, while you eat right, ensure you also exercise for at least an hour a day. Does that seem like a difficult thing to do? Well, the most common form of exercise is brisk walking.

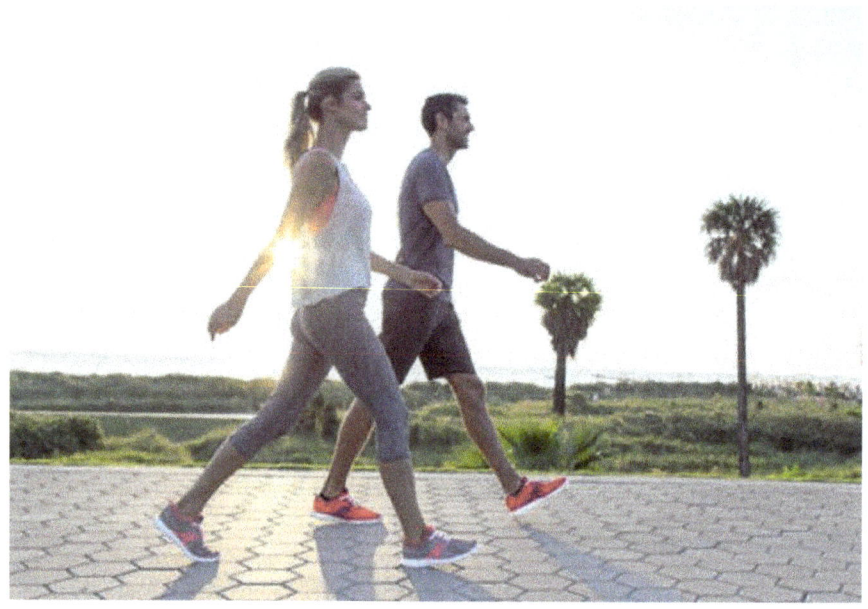

If you can increase the pace, going from walking to jogging, then you can still have some time at your disposal. You might need up to forty to forty-five minutes of exercise each day to maintain healthy body weight. It is important to recall that everyone's need is different. While some people need more training to shed weight, others require only a bit. The best way of moving away from the motionless lifestyle that characterizes the lives of many AFib patients is to get up and about.

Less Stress

Life is complicated, right? Telling yourself not to worry is not always enough in reality. Things can get tricky. They can get tough, and it sometimes seems like nothing is working. Suffering is said by some religious experts to be innate to life. All these factors usually combined manifest as stress. And as cute as that term sounds, there's nothing desirable about it.

A recent study has revealed that the effect of severe stress is as chaotic as smoking five cigarettes in a day. That's in correlation with another study which indicated that a lot of stress is enough to cut a person's life short by as much as ten years. It shouldn't come as a surprise, then, to learn that stress is a significant cause of atrial fibrillation. Even research has shown that stress and anxiety can increase the risk of developing AFib by fourfold.

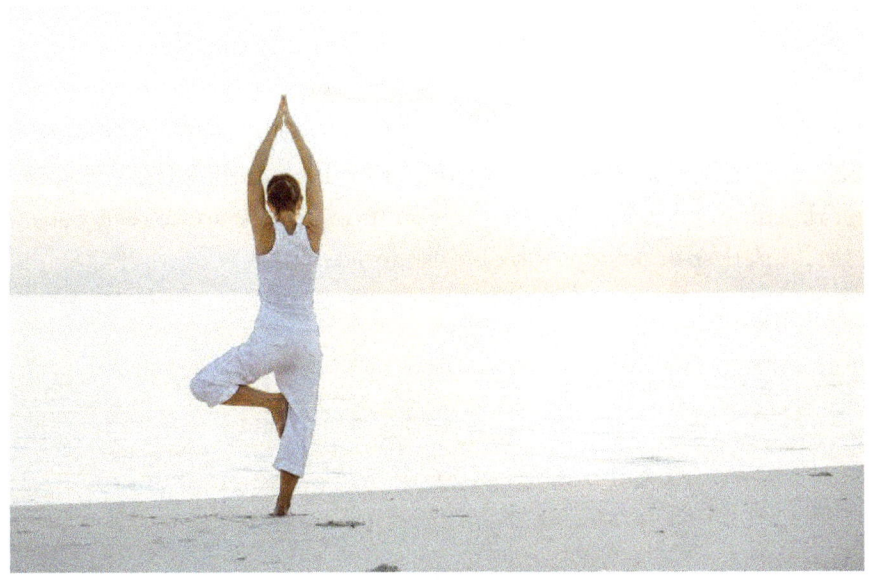

But if you can't put up with it, how do you address it?

Well, for beginners, you need to take an efficient approach to address the issues of stress. Moreover, it will enable you to reach your goal as timely as possible. So, what are some of these practical approaches? Let's take a look at them together.

- **Reassess Work**

When Swedish researchers reviewed the research establishing the connection between AFib and work stress, they came across findings that should motivate anyone suffering from the adverse effects of work stress to pay close attention. The review also established that individuals who experienced damaging work-related stress were more vulnerable to developing atrial fibrillation by 37 percent. That's quite huge. The worse part of the findings of this review was that women were found to be more susceptible to the risks of AFib. It was discovered that female workers who were victims of negative stress at work had a massive 79 percent risk of having AFib.

You need to ensure that you are not overworking yourself. If need be, delegate work and responsibilities to others in the office. If your work isn't flexible enough to give you time to have some rest, you should perhaps consider looking for another job.

- **Reconsider Stress**

Next time you find yourself standing in a long queue at the grocery store, or you're stuck in heavy traffic, or you're waiting for a friend who refused to show up at a meeting at the scheduled time, you should consider your emotional state. Why's this necessary? Because research has shown that the risk of an AFib attack is much more remarkable when you are feeling impatient. By estimates, it goes as far as threefold.

Lack of patience is one of the numerous emotions associated with life's negative stressors. While it is not just a necessity but a vital thing to reduce the potency of these stressors, the truth is that just a relatively low number of people have control over their circumstances, schedules, and surroundings. Sometimes, a physician's plan can run late. Sometimes, planes can get delayed. And sometimes, co-workers may fail to get their works done, and we are often affected. So, what do you do about situations like these that you have little or no power over?

You shouldn't be surprised that people who gave reports of high-stress levels in their daily lives were more likely to have health problems and die untimely. The significant part of this was that the reverse was the case with people who didn't view their stress as inimical to their wellbeing. It was as if their perception of stress made them immune to bad health outcomes. Thus, it would help if you perceived stress from a different angle. That's what this entails.

So, how do you change your perception of stress? You can do that by taking the pressure away. Do you remember the Prof. Reinhold Niebuhr Serenity Prayer, which reads, "God, give me the serenity to accept the things I cannot change, the courage to change the things I can, and the wisdom to know the difference"? This can be helpful. If you also believe that more stress in your life is beneficial, you'll likely birth a new perception about stress. Scientifically, the term "hormesis" means that a dose of different stressors can incite a pleasant biological response. With restrictions, it is even true that "what doesn't kill you makes you stronger."

When you constantly remind yourself that some stress is beneficial, and remember that whether good or bad, there are parts of your life that you can't always control; stress loses its strength to ruin your life.

- **Manage your Media Habits**

News can come in different doses. Sometimes, it can be good, and other times it can be harmful. This news triggers certain emotions in different individuals. The news which incites anger, for instance, is likely to increase your risk of having AFib. Research has shown that the risk of developing atrial fibrillation rises by six times following an experience of anger.

Feelings of sadness and anxiety, which some people already have in their lives, are often triggered by negative news. The chances of medical problems become higher with this. But how do you deal with this? Well, you can reduce your AFib risks by simply getting rid of news and social media. This doesn't mean that you should deprive yourself of the happenings around you. Instead, you can set up a schedule for going through the news. You can set aside every morning and evening to listen to the latest news, see sport updates, and watch celebrity gossip. When you have a fixed time for this, your stress will be put into remission.

Put an End to Smoking and Vaping

Smoking cigarettes is linked to many adverse health conditions; it's usually hard to keep the figures. There's stroke and coronary heart disease, colorectal cancer, stomach cancer, and lung cancer. In addition, there's chronic obstructive pulmonary disease, diabetes, and arthritis. So it shouldn't come as a surprise to know that smoking and AFib have a well-established connection. The lungs and the heart are delicately connected. Once one is polluted, the other also gets polluted. Not that anyone should need another reason to stop smoking, but if you've been diagnosed with AFib and you still smoke, your chances of putting AFib into remission is not feasible.

Let's talk about the other one. While many perceive vapes or e-cigarettes as "less bad" for their health than smoking, the reverse might be the case. Research has shown that e-cigarettes can be as harmful as traditional cigarettes, although in some different ways. The short-term and long-term effects of the chemicals used in making most of these vaping products are yet to be known. But the widespread knowledge, as mentioned earlier, is that both the lungs and heart are delicately connected, and any harm on one will result in the injury of the other. In addition, once the heart is affected, an enlargement in the heart chamber is induced, which results in irregular heart rhythm.

Yet, for many AFib patients, even those who know how detrimental vaping can be to their health, and those who are very aware of the connection between smoking and heart issues, quitting feel addictive. And without a shadow of doubt, it is difficult to stop.

Let's be frank here, no matter what you are doing to improve your health if you do not quit smoking, you don't stand a chance to see any remarkably positive impacts on your AFib. Most smokers have tried to stop. Some of them want to quit. Those who have been able to do so need several attempts to do so. If you're going to break the habit of smoking, it is mostly advised that you work hand in hand with your doctor, who can prescribe drugs that will help you break the cycle of addiction and take part in addiction-specific counselling.

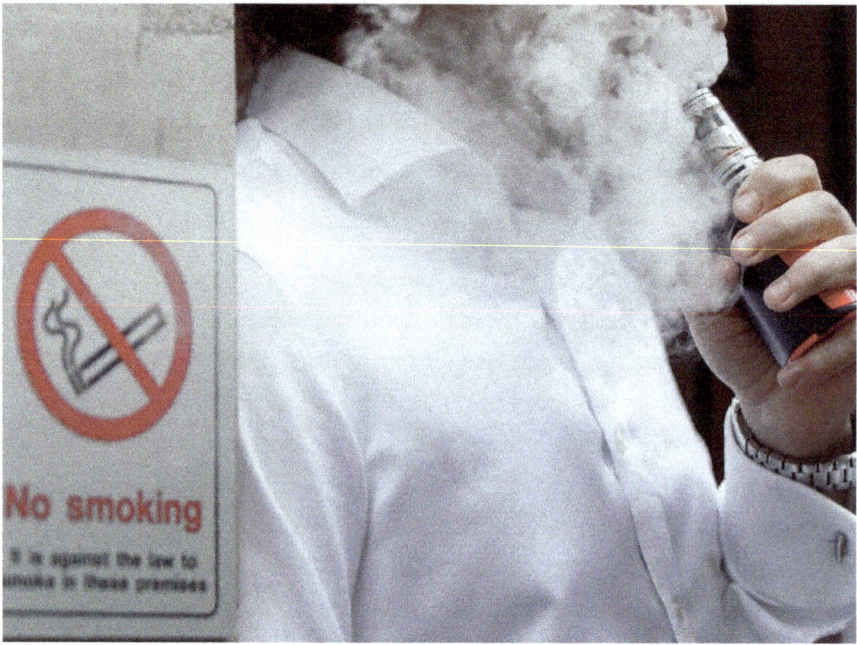

Putting an end to smoking comes with a lot of benefits. Not only does it reduce the risk of AFib, but it also reduces the risk of other diseases that can exacerbate atrial fibrillation or make it more challenging to address. You will also find it easier to breathe, particularly during exercise, if you quit smoking.

Chapter Three

Ablation: Why You Should Consider Ablation

Diagnosed with atrial fibrillation when he was in his mid-forties, Smith wasn't pleased with the idea that drugs were going to solve his problems. And to some extent, he was correct. To lose some weight, he started exercising every day and made the paleo diet his favourite. He adopted yoga to put stress into remission. Whenever he would have an attack of AFib, irrespective of where he found himself at the time, he would put an end to what he was doing and talk a brisk walk.

He adopted all these procedures, and they worked pretty well for him for a relatively long time.

Year after year, the one mild status of his AFib deteriorated rapidly, and even the procedures weren't offering the solutions he desired. Even the drugs weren't helping to keep his heart in rhythm. The following prescription that came from his doctor was amiodarone. Given the many adverse effects attached to this antiarrhythmic, Smith recognized a "no go area." No other option was available now but ablation.

Considering ablation is an option doesn't mean that you weren't good enough at following lifestyle optimization procedures. Likewise, it doesn't mean you weren't efficient in curing your AFib via other means. For example, even athletes diagnosed with AFib who are in the picture of health often resort to having AFib ablated after many aspects of their lives have been optimized and after medications have failed to produce a healthy outcome. Since many aspects of their lives have been optimized, they can go back to their physical activities, and competitions, without any drugs and any episodes of atrial fibrillation.

Catheter ablation

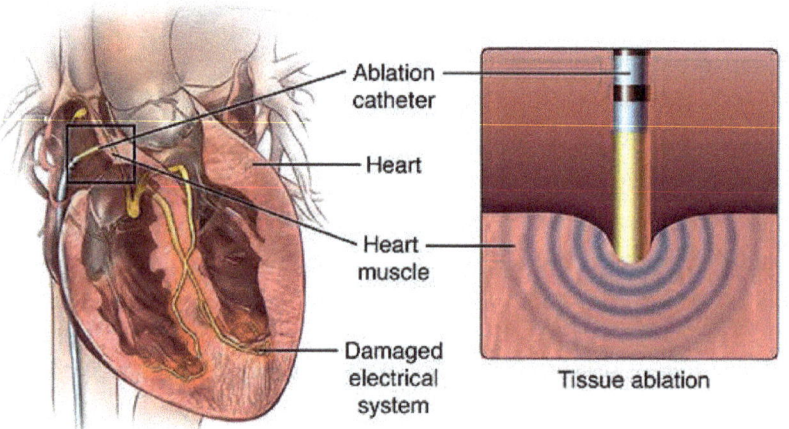

It can't be overemphasized: ablation isn't what you resort to after all other options have proven to be abortive. Ablation is a procedure that can be avoided with an aggressive and early lifestyle optimization, and it's nothing to be hasty about. Still, it's a necessary treatment for many people who require thorough discussion with an expert EP at no later time.

This was the option Smith settled for. And that was what gave him the health and life he had long desired.

During catheter ablation, an electrophysiologist (commonly referred to as an EP) controls the movement of many catheters- specially designed tools for working in the heart that is slowly inserted into a patient's body through a big inner thigh vein or sometimes through a neck vein. Many people still find it hard to believe that the human heart can be easily reached this way. But the practice of cardiac catheterization has been in existence for more than a century. The first of its kind was completed by Werner Forssmann, a German physician, who inserted a twenty-four-inch catheter through his arm to his right ventricular sinus in 1929. In past decades, doctors have moved catheters towards bad heart cells located in the atria. Those cells are damaged by either cryo energy (sometimes referred to as 'fires' and 'iced') or radiofrequency, thereby making a barrier of scar tissue to hinder abnormal electrical impulses from inducing AFib (such as electrically separating heart tissues close to the pulmonary vein), or directly destroying misfiring cells in the heart. Either way, the goal is to stop atrial fibrillation from resurfacing. In addition, since no cutting or stitching is required, patients can often return home quickly afterwards.

The process creates a kind of electrical bypass which removes bad heart cells. Therefore, the electrical charges that run through the heart of a patient have no other choice than to go through the other healthy tissues. Or, in much simpler terms, the electrical charges have no means of going through the bad cells. Studies have shown that as long as these bad cells have been eliminated, the rest of the heart, including the atria and the ventricles, become much stronger since they now work together in unison.

The outcome seems like a miracle. Patients who had had all hopes dashed with several cardioversions, medications, and hospitalizations are instantly freed from their problems.

But this is unlike a miracle. It is a medical process- and a serious one at that. And if it all you want to adopt this procedure, you should get yourself acquainted with as much information as possible about the policies.

The Procedures

The night before ablation is carried out, the patients are advised to stay away from food and water until the process is completed. It's more like a fast. Several days before the procedure is carried out, patients are often advised to discontinue taking rate-controlling drugs, but this should be done concerning the doctor's directives. Contrarily, most EPs will have you continue using your rate-controlling drugs (anticoagulants).

Once you get to the hospital, you will change into a gown and meet with a staff of hospital workers and medical personnel who will be on the ground for the procedures, and the anesthesiologist and the electrophysiologist.

Some ablations are carried out under traditional anesthesia and sedation. This process is called conscious sedation, whereby the patient is awake but drowsy while other ablations are carried out under general anesthesia. Here, the patient is completely asleep and uses a respirator or breathing tube during the procedure. Unlike in Asia and Europe, where conscious sedation is commonly practiced, perhaps due to the scarcity of an anesthesiologist in large numbers, general anesthesia is common in the United States. There are none of these two procedures that don't have their advantages and disadvantages. During general anesthesia, you are completely asleep and sedentary. It allows the 3D maps designed to find the parts of the heart that require treatment to be more accurate. Also, it is a calm working atmosphere for your EPs, as they can focus solely on the seat without having to bother about their patients waking up while the procedure is going on. However, the disadvantage of this procedure is that the initial twenty-four hours of recovery can be quite tricky.

Before the procedure starts, each catheter- possibly one in the neck and multiple in the inner thigh- must be inserted into a vein through a small sheath, usually a more extended and larger IV that holds the vein firmly open so the catheter can move in and out of the vein without any obstruction.

Once all these catheters have entered the heart of the patient, the EP sets out to work. AFib triggers are most commonly on the left side of the heart, while the catheters are placed into the veins on the right side of the heart. To get to the right atrium, the catheters are moved via a thin tissue (called the septum) into the left atrium. The cavity created by this closes 3 to 4 weeks after completion of the procedure. Next, the EP progresses to map out the parts of the hearts that need to be treated, add part-by-part radiofrequency energy to separate the pulmonary veins, and treat any "bad area." If, on the other hand, the EP chooses to use a cryoballoon, the mapping process will likely be skipped, and the pulmonary veins will electrically be separated using a cryoballoon. As a result of the heavy size of the cryoballoon, it is often difficult to treat any other arrhythmia. If present, more catheters are required to do the mapping and ablating of these areas.

Does this sound like a demanding process? Of course, it is. Even with the most advanced technology at disposal, the procedure of ablation is a patient and meticulous one. Healthy and unhealthy parts of tissues are interwoven in a minimal closure, being moved here and there by blood flow and contradictions of the heart. As a result of this, it takes time. Catheter ablation can last about two hours, or even four hours, depending on how complicated the condition of the person's heart is, the experience level of the EP, and the complexities of the treatment.

Once catheters have been removed and the procedure is completed, the patient will be monitored while he gradually comes out of anesthesia. More often than not, younger and healthier patients are allowed to return home the same day, while others might be advised to stay until the next day. This largely depends on the principles of treatment put in place by the hospital. It varies from hospital to hospital.

The procedures discussed here encompass the general processes of any ablation. But, that doesn't mean that there aren't other ways of going about it.

When All Else Fails

No one newly diagnosed with atrial fibrillation or has recently learned that he is at risk of having AFib goes without making a profound resolution to take the necessary steps to put the disease into remission through an optimized lifestyle. It is also the safest and best approach and the most adopted approach by those who have chosen to read this book.

It does not mean that this technique works for everyone. Some people can try a combination of balanced metabolism, better and quality sleep, lack of negative work stress, and avoiding polluted environment, including smoking and vaping; often, it is not enough to put all of their AFib-induced biomarkers into remission. It wasn't that these techniques couldn't work; perhaps because of one reason or the other, they couldn't adhere strictly to every one of these approaches without making mistakes along the way. Irrespective of how committed they were to fight against the disease; they end up going back to their previous lifestyle. Biomarkers that have risen to a significantly healthy level indicating a healthy heart begins to decline. The greatest biomarker of all: weight gradually goes up. And like before, their heart begins to sway away.

It is at this point that they resort to ablation. And it is instantly after this procedure that patients always feel like they have been injected with another potent dose of energy.

You must ensure that these moments aren't in vain. First, you should be aware that what ablation does is fix your present misfiring atrial fibrillation circuit. It has little or no role to play in preventing the future occurrence of an attack. Thus, to avoid ever undergoing another ablation procedure, you have to adopt practical approaches to address the substrate causes of your AFib. Honestly, there have been cases of significantly overweight people who have undergone ablation without suffering a future attack of the disease, but this is by far an exception. An ablation is a reset, an opportunity to give your heart a new beginning. Thus, if you have been waiting for it, here it is.

It was the same opportunity Debbie had and using it, she was able to beat AFib at its game. She had done well to make her sleep a top priority, having at least seven hours of sleep per night and ensuring that she had enough rest. In addition, she reduced the stress, sought a cleaner and healthier environment, and exercised more.

"And when it finally came to taking those last few steps, particularly concerning my choice of food, I felt very vulnerable," she said. "I was conversant with the steps; how to go about my daily exercise, how to avoid processed and fast foods, yes, I knew everything. But there was always this feeling of fatigue that I think could have been due to the drugs I was taking. So the more tired I got, the less the strength I had to go outside for exercise. Even worse, my choice of food wasn't healthy at all, and even when I tried to make a healthy choice, there wasn't any significant reduction in my weight. Well, it could have been due to the drugs I was on".

However, there was a turnaround after she had her ablation.

"Some days after the procedure, I was still feeling some pain. However, weeks followed, and I didn't notice any episode of AFib. Although I hadn't gotten all the energy I had before the ablation procedure, yet it happened sooner than expected".

She felt the strength, the energy. The time to walk, to run, to exercise was now there. She could breathe well; her lungs were filled with air and her heart with joy. And with that same vibe, she knew she could win the long-term fight against obesity.

This was a moment of confidence after the ablation procedure. Debbie summoned her family together and sought their permission to make some healthy decisions, particularly for her sake. She asked if they could, devote themselves to 90 percent of unprocessed foods with no sugar. She knew how indispensable exercise was and, for that reason, pleaded to her family to make the gym a regular place to visit. Normal, brisk walking and bike cycling, perhaps after dinner every night, was also recommended.

Although challenging, yet she had to make those decisions. "Some came with tears," she recalled. "I had to push all my family into it to make sure that it was easy for me. And I was so glad when they all consented to do everything in their capacity to help me reach that goal. It was much more out of love and concern for one another".

The truth is, there might not be anything magical about cycling, or walking, or visiting the gym with members of your family, monitoring your diets closely to avoid taking processed and fast foods with sugar. But, contrarily, these are procedures associated with a balanced metabolism that are specific, measurable, achievable, realistic, and timely - otherwise called SMART goals.

Conclusion – Part 2

Why You Should Stop The Use of Unnecessary Medications

Like Flora, several AFib patients are often advised to "stop taking X and start using Y." But you must be sure that you are doing the right thing, and that goes to your doctor as well. Failure to know which medications to use and when to use them, particularly on the part of the physician, will likely leave the scar untreated. Although there's always a gradual shift in treatment paradigms, and that's a good thing.

So, to many people, especially those who for the first time suffered atrial fibrillation, the advice Flora got: take medication, is perceived as the right advice. However, the substrate causes that induced her AFib had been there many years, developing and spreading their tentacles across every part of the heart. That means that if she wanted to treat the condition, she needed enough time to confront AFib and the entire substrate causes. And this can only be achieved by taking meds.

However, medications are a two-edged sword. For one benefit, there can be a large number of adverse effects attached.

The good news, however, is that most of these side effects are well known. Creating drugs from production to the development processes, up and until approval of the FDA in the United States can last for as long as ten years. During this period, the medications are rigorously tested and examined before they are released into the medicine cabinets to be used by patients across the length and breadth of the country. (Similar schedules and timelines are adopted by other national and international regulatory bodies such as the European Agency for the Evaluation of Medicinal Products). Once drugs are used across the country, the length of likely side effects can be easily ascertained. Since almost all of the most popular AFib medications have been FDA-approved about ten years ago, any bad thing associated with them has likely been noted.

It is a natural feeling, and this is common with everyone when you get worried about using medications that are said to have adverse side effects. And this is one of the primary reasons why many people suffering from atrial fibrillation are shifting from drugs to supplements. However, the problem with supplements is that there are no industries responsible for regulating them. And since there are no regulatory bodies, the content of these supplements is not often disclosed.

To be candid, taking drugs and supplements is difficult. The biological purposes they are created to achieve are far too hard and essential for that effect not to be felt in organs elsewhere in a user's body. In addition, a large number of genetic and epigenetic X components are too many to account for all of them. It means that just a little out of the many AFib patients will find the right drugs and supplements that restore the standard of life they truly desire.

So, as far as AFib drugs are concerned, there is a wide margin of bad news about them. And you must consider this awful news before using any medication. Thus, you must understand the procedures and everything about drugs because the other procedures unveiled in the subsequent chapters of this book might be pretty challenging to follow.

But if you choose to adhere strictly to these procedures, you will likely end up with a drug-free solution to your condition. However, before you can have a good understanding of these other procedures, you must be acquainted with drugs prescribed to atrial fibrillation patients.

INTRODUCTION – PART 3

Tracking Wellness

Remember when you used to keep track of the time using a watch? Wasn't that all that was required? Even then, you could keep track of your heart health by using a powerful device called a timepiece. But, first, you needed to check your heartbeat rate to locate your pulse, count your heartbeats for 15 seconds, and multiply what you got by 4.

Tracking other pieces of data, including the rate of your heartbeats during exercise and the speed of your heartbeats while resting, can be a significant venture. You don't necessarily need to go through all this stress to have your beats tracked today. A smartwatch can combine all of these features and give you the most accurate data that you need. It doesn't end there. A smartwatch is also efficient at helping people detect atrial fibrillation.

When Shaw got his first EKG smartwatch (approved by the FDA), he didn't get it for the atrial fibrillation features. He liked it because he was a big fan of Apple devices. He got the Apple Watch 4.

But he should be grateful he did. The year before he got the smartwatch, he noticed some decline in strength and energy, which reduced the amount of exercise he was getting. "Initially, I had thought it was one of the signs that I wasn't on the good side of age anymore," he said. "The good days were always there, and the bad days weren't editable. So that's a sign you are getting old, right?"

Within a couple of days, he thought he would be able to get back into shape through the apps on his smartwatch that helped him keep track of his exercise and walks. But it wasn't long after he got the watch that he was notified of some arrhythmia. Since it hadn't happened to him before, he was less concerned. However, it soon became apparent to him that his condition was a potential risk for a much more devastating condition. At that point, he had no other option than to see his family doctor, who then referred him to a cardiologist in a nearby hospital. After an EKG, the doctor confirmed that Shaw had atrial fibrillation, prescribed the usual drugs, and sent him away.

Nevertheless, Shaw kept getting AFib alerts. "And this time, it became more and more serious," he uttered. "The watch had been right all the while, but I didn't take it seriously. It had warned me of a potential arrhythmia, and certainly, that was what the doctor diagnosed. So when it became pronounced that the meds weren't keeping my heart in rhythm as the case had been, I was frightened".

He could have done nothing at that point; he had to pay his cardiologist a second visit. After relating his experiences to the cardiologist, he knew that it was high time he referred him (Shaw) to an EP.

Just imagine this: because Shaw's symptoms were so intermittent and subtle, he would probably not have known that he was suffering from atrial fibrillation for several months, if not years. But, as luck would have it, the smartwatch helped him detect his AFib, and that made it possible for his condition to be treated early, long before it deteriorates into atrial fibrosis. Therefore, it isn't an overstatement to say that Shaw's smartwatch saved him the stress of suffering a worse nightmare like an AFib stroke.

Now to a lot of people, an AFib-detecting smartwatch may not be necessary. They think every episode of atrial fibrillation can be felt.

However, even research has shown that many people with atrial fibrillation experience episodes that can't be felt. So what's worse than waiting for an episode of atrial fibrillation to become so strong and evident that it can be felt? That could mean more harm to your health and whole life.

Further research has indicated that symptoms perceived to be AFib-related a 50 percent chance of being something else to make things worse. Moreover, to make things even more complicated, if you had at one point or another undergone AFib ablation, plenty of the cardiac nerves that initially helped you feel your AFib symptoms might have also been corrected as part of the procedure. Thus, there is no evidence as to whether your symptoms will still clearly show future episodes of atrial fibrillation.

These factors combined are why having a smartwatch to detect your AFib episodes is indispensable.

Recall, atrial fibrillation is often irregular and fast rhythm- so much such that detecting the pattern of the beats isn't always easy. This rule isn't familiar to everyone, though. There have been many cases of AFib patients who had very slow heartbeats with their atrial fibrillation. So, don't rule out its chance of being AFib just because your heart isn't beating fast.

Remember the second type of arrhythmia: atrial flutter? This one is always regular and fast with a persistent and patterned beat. However, like atrial fibrillation, this can also come without being fast, but you hardly see cases of this.

Premature beats? Yes, that's another one. Examples include premature ventricular contractions and premature atrial contractions. They cause a normal to somewhat less heart rate but with a distinct pattern to the irregularity. For instance, you may have four to five regular beats, and then one or two beat(s) that is/are off.

Do you necessarily need to know all these? Isn't that what the smartwatch is supposed to do?

Although there is an improvement on these watches, and some producers claim up to 100 percent accuracy, there have been cases where even top-of-the-chart AFib-detecting smartwatches failed to offer the correct diagnosis.

There are many benefits you can get from these devices, particularly concerning putting your AFib into remission and keeping it there. Therefore, in the subsequent paragraphs of this section, we will be discussing the various parts of your life that can be easily tracked using a smartwatch: sleep, stress, exercise, and several others.

Tracking Sleep

When you get up from bed in the morning, what's the first thing that you do? Do you reach out for the TV remote and click on the news? Do you reach out for your mobile phone? Or do you kiss your partner?

What's usually the last thing you do when you go to bed at night? Do you have a drink? Do you click on the TV news to see the wrap of the day's activities? Or you pray and go to bed?

Whatever the habits that you have cultivated to guide your wake-and-sleep lifestyle, there is another one you need to add, in fact, a couple of them. As part of your first and last actions of the day, you should endeavor to track your sleep constantly.

Let's begin from the end of the day. What time do you often go to bed? You ate, sure aware that going to bed does not mean that you are going to sleep. After getting to bed, some group of people usually grab a novel and run through the pages. Between the period that the light finally goes off and the time you're gradually drifting to sleep, there are a couple of other things that can happen. But, having a record of your bedtime, with accuracy, allows you to understand better the medium by which you sleep.

Then, the following day when you wake up from sleep, you should note the quality and quantity of REM sleep you had. Unfortunately, the earlier apps designed to record REM sleep amounts were not accurate and reliable enough. However, today, many programs and devices are better prepared to get more accurate data and are, without a doubt, worth using, as REM is a strong indicator of better quality sleep, which correlates with AFib. Generally, REM sleep should account for as much as 50 percent of the sleep you have every night.

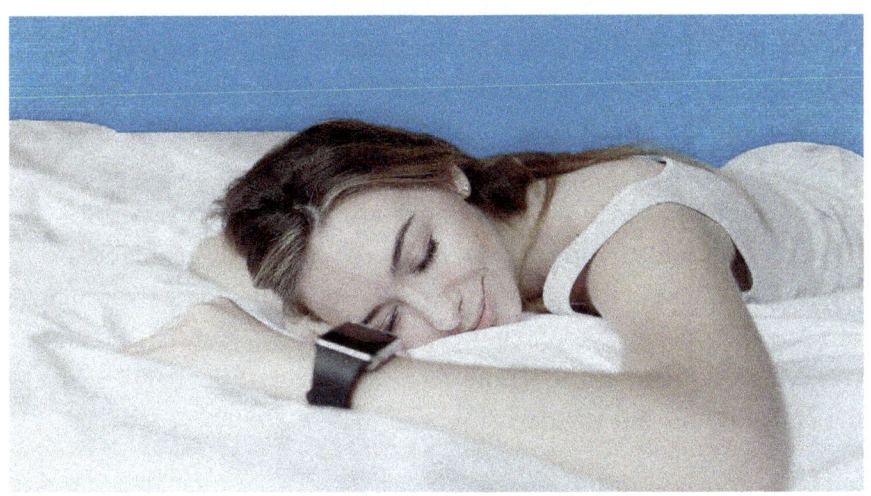

Looking at the figures isn't enough. You need to ensure that a log to which you can refer from time to time is kept. Without that, it won't be easy to know if you are improving or not. You will even find it harder to observe the nuances that can assist people not only to reduce bit also to eliminate every risk of AFib episodes.

Once you've noted those significant figures, which are objective measures, it might be perfect for penning down some notes about your sleep. For example, was it an alarm that woke you up? Or you woke up naturally? Well, you should have at this point know that the goal of every procedure or step in this book is for long-term benefit. The long-term goal is to wake up naturally. If this happens seldomly, it is evidence that you need to reconsider your bedtime as well as other factors militating against your sleep.

Moreover, did you have to wake up in the middle of the night? Did you have to get up to use the restroom? Do you think your evening fluid consumption might have been responsible for the restroom visits? Have you observed any connection between evening exercise and the quality of your sleep? Do you think this exercise may reduce the number of times you wake up at night to use the restroom? Do you think this exercise may as well make you have a better sleep? Do you find it difficult to go to sleep early due to the bulky emails you have to respond to? Or maybe your work assignments are delaying your sleep? Do TV programs after dinner affect bedtime or the ease with which you fall asleep? Were you having regular nightmares that correlate with when you started taking a particular drug or personal stressor? All these are subjective factors, and since you are the subject of the whole thing, the level of the data highly depends on you and the decisions you make.

Tracking Stress

Stress is one of the most evident triggers for atrial fibrillation. However, it is also a subjective metric. It is because what is emotionally and mentally stressful to an individual might not be stressful to another. In addition, whatever is making you feel stressed today isn't likely to make you feel the same way the next day. More so, you shouldn't be worried about emotional and mental stress alone; physical stress can also induce an episode of atrial fibrillation.

However, by tracking the variability of your heart rate or by HRV, you can get an accurate measure of the amount of all types of stress that is felt by your heart. Even studies have indicated that the higher your HRV figures, the lower your risk of developing an episode of AFib. Of course, even when your heart is in perfect sinus rhythm, some beat-to-beat variability is inevitable.

With the aid of a smartwatch, you can now take accurate measurements of your HRV; however, you must have it in mind that studies have indicated that such measures should be done manually to ascertain the accuracy of the test. The perfunctory HRV recordings that continue to go on in the background while you go about your daily activities are unreliable.

So, what HRV figure should you aim for? Among the different measurements of HRV available, the best studied probably is the standard deviation of beat-to-beat variability, which are often referred to as N to N interviews, and for that reason, the name SDNN. Your risks of having a heart attack, arrhythmia, or dying go down significantly when your SDNN is above 50 milliseconds. Therefore, ideally, you should aim big at something above 100 milliseconds. For example, one research revealed that maintaining an HRV over 100 milliseconds reduces the risk of dying by fivefold.

A single figure won't do you the good that you need. Thus, you need to track the statistics over time. That will enable you to know the rate at which stress wax and wane from one day to another. If your HRV is continuously running low, what that means is that your heart is perhaps crushed from excess mental, emotional, or physical stress.

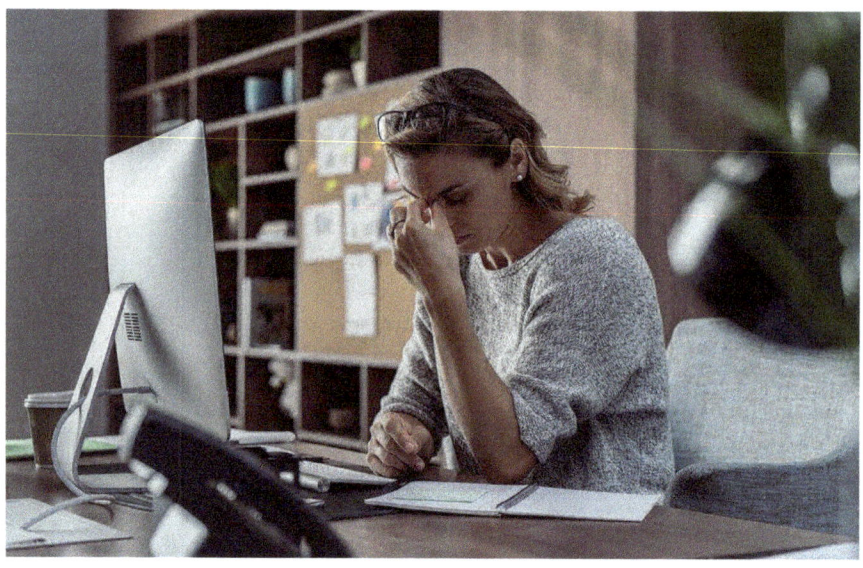

For instance, if you are not sleeping well, or you're being stressed at work, or you're making very unhealthy food choices, or you aren't getting enough exercise as you should, then the level of your HRV will below. And when that happens (when your HRV is low), you're more vulnerable to heart attack, atrial fibrillation, injuries, and illnesses. Frankly, perpetually low HRV recordings have been revealed to indicate future episodes of AFib even as much as fifteen years into the future.

However, an HRV that is running high tells you that your heart is giving the proper response to the emotional, physical, and mental stress that characterizes your daily life. As a result, your heart is happy, and your life is not out of balance.

You should be aware that your HRV number is expected to be falsely elevated by arrhythmias. An accurate HRV measurement cannot be obtained during premature ventricular contractions, premature atrial contractions, atrial flutter, or atrial fibrillation. So, for this test to be carried out, your heart must be in normal sinus rhythm void of excess premature beats.

Tracking Exercise

There are several means of going about this. But the best thing might be to take a step, then take another action, and then another, and ensure that your phone or smartwatch does the recording as you go.

Tracking your steps as you take them is one healthy way research has proven to get your health to balance. But, unfortunately, it's also one part of your life that's likely the most difficult to fudge, and that's pretty interesting because studies have revealed that more and more people are often not sincere with themselves about the amount of exercise they are getting- conspicuously overestimating the amount of activity they get, the amount of time they spend while exercising, and the vigor of the exercise.

Vigor is indispensable. This is why it is not usually enough to take many steps each day, even if you walk throughout the day. At some point, you may also reach the end of diminishing returns. That's why it is also vital that you use your phone or smartwatch to track the number of calories you burn day after day. The estimated amount of burnt calories displayed by these devices might not be so accurate. Not everyone is the same. Nevertheless, whatever figure your smartwatch/phone displays will be derived the same way tomorrow as today, and the same way yesterday as today. You have nothing to worry about.

What the figures show, is a general overview of what you have been doing overtime. Notwithstanding, it is not a bad thing if you keep personal details such as your age, gender, weight, height, and several other factors; up to date on the smartwatch/phone to improve the accuracy of the multiple algorithms.

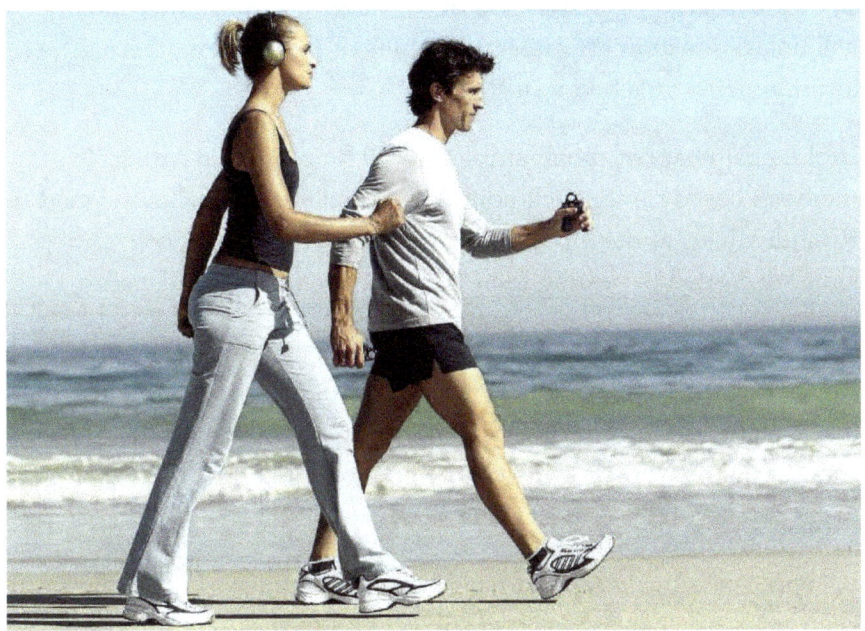

In a similar vein, indicating to your device the type of exercise you are doing, take, for instance, walking, running, or cycling can significantly make the activity tracking much more accurate.

Tracking Food

Of course, you can't wake up each day without putting something in your mouth. And unlike other factors that have been discussed, which require little effort (just with the aid of a smartwatch) to track, tracking food can be pretty demanding. However, irrespective of how demanding the process of tracking food and other factors will be examined in the later paragraphs of this section, there are a lot of benefits attached to it.

In the next chapter, much emphasis will be placed on eating methods based on the well-conducted research, specially designed for individuals at risk of AFib, or who have AFib, or those who have succeeded in putting their AFib into remission and want to keep it there.

But as mentioned in the previous part, just any food that helps you lose weight and keep it off without having any adverse side effects on other parts of your body can be an integral part of the procedures to fight against AFib.

Irrespective of what type of food you eat or how you eat, failure to keep track of what you eat will subject you to making unhealthy food decisions that would have been avoided if you had an accurate account of your eating. Even worse, you'll likely miss out on a lifetime opportunity to build and maintain a heart rhythm that will help you understand and control your condition. The impacts that a poor/bad meal, for instance, will have on the psychological and physical wellbeing of a specific individual will be quite different from its effects on another individual. Of course, this doesn't mean that you should intentionally choose to make unhealthy food decisions. Still, most people have limited willpower, and there's the presence of a significant currency that will help you to know the foods that will likely affect your weight, AFib attacks, amongst other biomarkers. And you don't want to learn that stuff without tracking, do you?

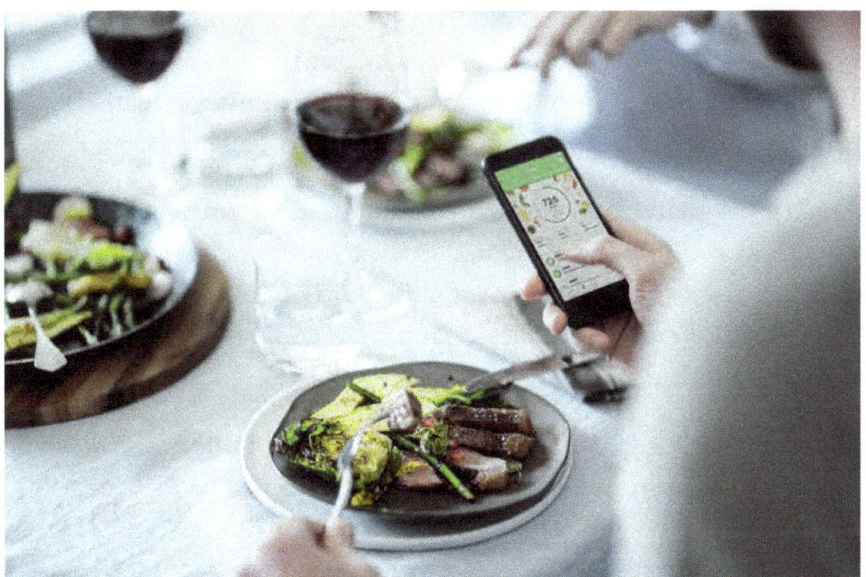

Now, food tracking isn't the same as counting calories.

For some group of people, counting calories comes with accountability and awareness. And that's OK. However, calories, first conceived as a word in the mid-1800s and initially based on the amount of energy required to increase the temperature of one gram of water by one degree Celsius, are an imperfect measure of nutrition.

Not all calories are the same. It's easy to perceive this when you consider 100 calories. For instance, 100 calories of a processed cereal breakfast are guaranteed to raise your insulin and blood glucose levels in such a way that you will not feel full for as long as the cereal metabolically causes harm to your body. On the other hand, 100 calories of almonds will gear your body into action processing a group of nutrients that take several hours to break down, thereby keeping you metabolically active and healthy and makes you feel full far beyond that of processed foods. Even when taking natural, non-processed diets, a calorie differs from a calorie. Broccoli is different from fish, and fish is different from carrots. Carrots are also different from almonds. Do you grab the point?

The truth is that people generally tend to underestimate significantly the number of calories contained in their foods and overestimate their burned calories. This way, the method of balancing metabolism is rendered useless. And what could be more complicated than this?

Here's the warning: if by counting the number of calories, you have been able to put your weight under check and maintain a very healthy body mass index, you should continue with the trend. Don't tamper with the success. What's more, you already know the basics surrounding food tracking; however, don't stop there; there is still a lot to learn.

What haven't you been keeping track of all along? Yes, your nutrients. If this were some ten or twenty years back, this would have been a "mission impossible" for many people. Generally, scientists believe that the human body needs two primary fatty minerals, fifteen minerals, thirteen vitamins, and nine amino acids of food to live. And that's still not all. Many other molecules are beneficial to human health, not to mention other unhealthy chemicals that are devastatingly inimical. It would take only a supercomputer to combine all the figures created by these chemicals together.

Today, though, what could have been considered a supercomputer some decades back can neatly fit into your purse or pocket? Also, apps specially designed to help tracking and balancing food choices are available in large numbers, inexpensive, and extensively user-friendly. All that is required of you is to open the app, type in the food name, and the computer takes it up from there.

Don't be surprised to learn that if there's any food substance you need to monitor or track, it must be fiber first. Why fiber? That's because fiber consumption from original food sources is a strong indicator of the quality of your food and your vulnerability to cardiovascular diseases. Research shows that you can reduce your risk of cardiovascular disease by one percent for each gram of fiber you consume daily above the stipulated amount (which is estimated at 30 grams per day). Sugar is another important thing you need to track. As far as this is concerned, the goal should be keeping it at a level as minimal as zero. That's quite an impossible feat. About 95 percent of what you eat daily contains sugar. Here's the thing that you should know: there's no health benefit derived from sugar consumption. Instead, this food substance poses many threats to your health and increases your risk of heart-related problems.

Apart from sugar and fiber, other nutrients you need to keep track of include other macronutrients like fat, carbohydrate, and protein. After monitoring this group, you can progress to track minerals and vitamins. These nutrients offer significant depth to the data. For example, with the aid of a nutrient-monitoring app, you can keep track of A, B12, C, and D, as well as iron, folate, zinc, and calcium.

Tracking Weight

Let's take a look at the biggest biomarker: your weight.

When asked what the best thing one can do to put one's AFib into remission, I respond by telling people to keep their weight at a relatively healthy level. However, as much as this is important, it is far more critical for you to track your weight day after day. Even how do you know you are overweight if you do not monitor the level of your weight?

Let's be clear on one thing: you have to track your weight every day. It can't be overemphasized enough. Your daily number will be one of the best predictors you'll get of the total impacts of all the other things you are doing to confront your atrial fibrillation.

Whatever the scale records are what it is, and this shouldn't cause any fear in you. Beating yourself up over records or lamenting about how far you still have to go isn't necessary. What will do you good, try as much as possible to monitor these records over time.

To keep track of your weight record, you can use WIFI- or Bluetooth-enabled smart scales. That's good, but considering all of the reasons discussed in the previous part of this book, you must know the usefulness of this record and the direction it is heading.

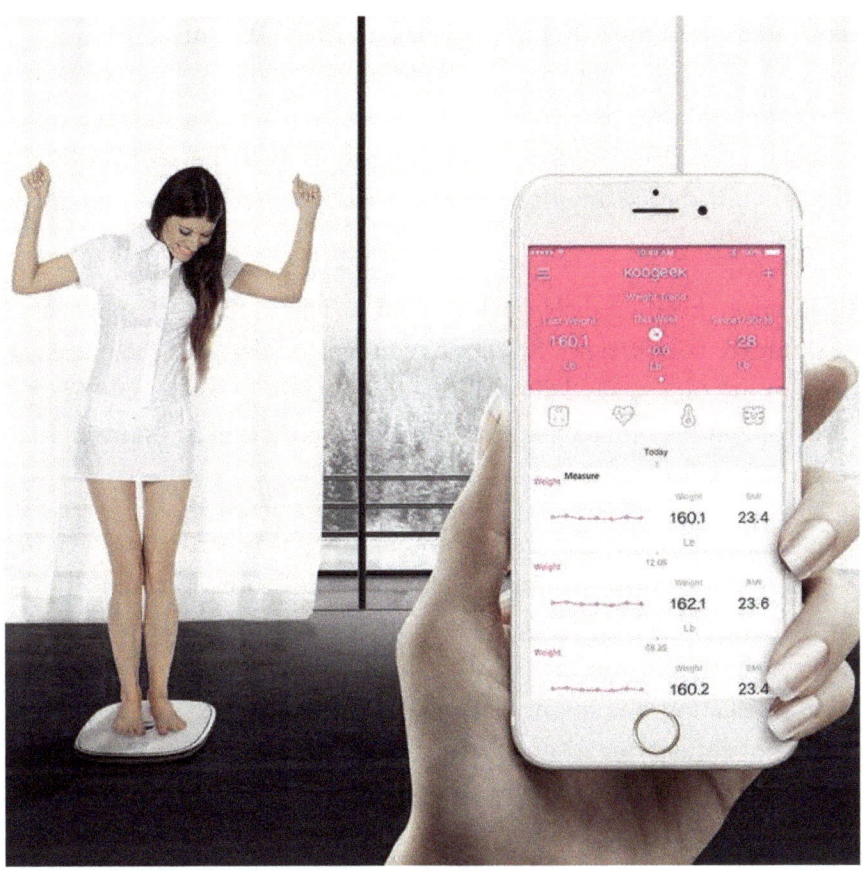

So, why can't you choose to track your weight monthly or at least when there's a need for it? Two reasons will be given here.

First and foremost, the simple act of stepping your feet on a scale to take a daily record of your weight can give you a significant boost of self-control because it affords you the opportunity for self-accountability, self-correction, and personal reflection. Will the simple knowledge that you will be stepping on a scale in less than 24 hours magically prevent you from grabbing a snack in a nearby restaurant during a work break or maneuvering your car to a city mall to get burger and fries when you are well disposed to the fact that carrots and nuts should be your favorite? Of course, not. However, it comes with a lot of benefits. Since decisions like these are made day after day, you should try to do all you can to give yourself immediate feedback and strength to make better health decisions. If there's anything you have to do to reduce your risk, you should do it.

In addition, keeping daily track of your weight is the best approach to optimize your weight. Studies have revealed that just the mere act of stepping on a scale daily reduces your weight by as much as threefold and is one of the most accurate predictors of that weight reduction.

Of course, not everyone with AFib has a problem with their weight. You'll remember, for example, that atrial fibrillation is common among athletes who engage in endurance sports, many of whom don't have weight problems. Also, many of those who suffer from atrial fibrillation due to familial genetic make-ups are lean. So, even if you have met your goal of balanced weight, you must cultivate the habit of checking your weight daily to avoid a sudden increase in weight that will further make you susceptible to AFib episodes.

Tracking Medications

Although, people who adopt the principles of lifestyle optimization long before their condition exacerbate won't ever have to start taking any AFib drug. Yet, doctors always tend to encourage their AFib patients to take medications at some point. And more often than not, that's the perfect advice. Drugs can be essential in some situations, mainly when your life and health are at stake.

As you work towards taking unnecessary meds, tracking your drugs isn't just going to be helpful; it will be indispensable, especially when you are already gradually approaching the minimal effective doses. Luckily, for you, tracking your medications isn't as demanding as monitoring food. You know why? While there are several food types, patients are only advised to take a few AFib drugs, and those meds are prescribed in specific dosages. So, as long as you use your drugs in the same way, it will be very much easier for you to see the effect of changes.

However, the big issue is that many people don't adhere to the doctor's instructions regarding using a drug. Once they forget to take the meds on one day, they will double it the next day. Even those who do well to take their meds every day don't do it at the exact hour every day. You might not be aware, but just a few hours play a very crucial role in how your body responds to drugs.

So, what do you do to address the situation? Just like tracking your sleep and exercise, a smartwatch can serve you right in this regard. Drug-monitoring apps with 'push reminders' can be pretty effective at helping you take the correct quantity of drugs daily, at the exact time every day. This will give you the chance to see and feel the actual impacts of those drugs in your daily, weekly, and even your monthly data.

Tracking Blood Pressure

In most the AFib-related research, it was discovered that a large percentage of AFib patients had high blood pressure as one of their atrial fibrillation risk factors. It shouldn't sound surprising to you since high blood pressure and its accomplice: hypertension, significantly increase the risk of having atrial fibrillation. Therefore, it makes a lot of sense to have this included in your tracking list.

There are two reasons you need to track your blood pressure. The first reason is quite apparent: you want to make sure that the level of your blood pressure doesn't rise so much so that it increases your risk of heart failure, atrial fibrillation, and other types of fibrosis. Secondly, as you optimize your lifestyle, it is very likely that (unless it's been years since you suffered high blood pressure) your high blood pressure will naturally go away, signifying that there is a significant improvement in your health. For those who are on blood pressure meds, it is also a great piece of information. There have been cases of various patients who didn't survive due to continuous use of blood pressure drugs even after their blood pressure had reduced considerably due to the healthy lifestyle they had adopted.

There are simple, inexpensive home-monitoring kits that you can use for that purpose to track your blood pressure. If you have one at your disposal, you can use it. Most times, you monitor your blood pressure when you are relaxed. Then, a few minutes after relaxation (say something like 5 minutes), with the cuff at the level of your heart or around your arm, you can take the measurement. If this first attempt fails to generate an accurate result, give it a space of three minutes and then try again. Make sure you track your blood pressure the same way each time.

There is another option you can choose to use: the blood pressure machine. Most people go for this option because the device is also good at detecting irregular pulses. As long as you continue checking from time to time, at least twice daily, you'll get accurate tracks of your blood pressure as well as your AFib. Whichever way you choose to go about it, tracking your blood pressure will help you make decisions to protect your health.

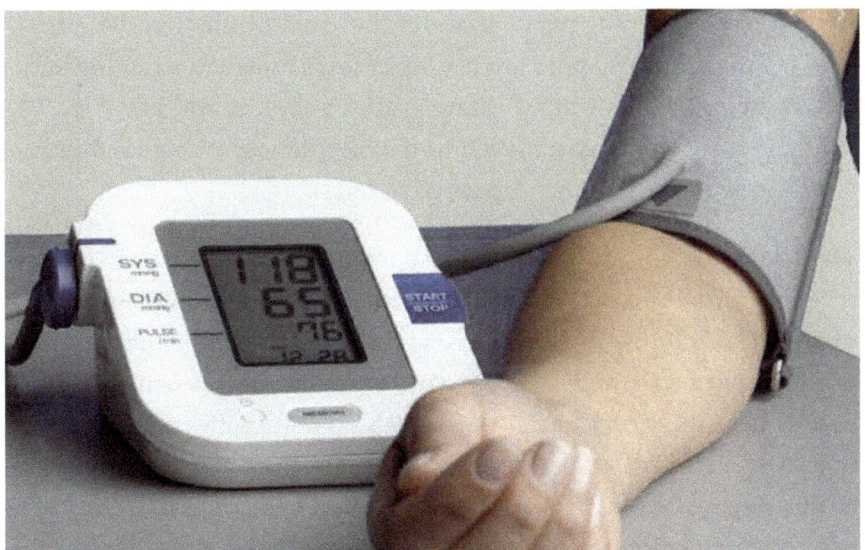

CHAPTER ONE:

THE AFIB DIET

If there's anything peculiar about the atrial fibrillation diet, then it's the fact that there are no restrictions attached to it. Rather than limits, this way of eating is about choices and lifestyle. Moreover, if you are committed to making the right choice of diet, you'll likely never feel the impact of hunger.

The beauty of this story is that these research-based diets are vital in reversing atrial fibrillation, usually without ablation procedure and meds. To reach that goal, though, you can't just change the way you eat. You have to change the way you live every day. When many people hear the word "diet," the first thing that comes to their mind is going on and off on a particular meal. But this isn't the case. Diet, in this sense, is a sophisticated lifestyle. You hold on to it and continue practicing for life. Failure to do it in a day will show that something is missing in your life. This is a lifestyle.

So, what's the purpose of this lifestyle? This lifestyle is specifically designed to counteract and mitigate the underlying factors that cause atrial fibrillation. It borders around how to eat (avoiding over-fullness, slow and steady, and keeping triggers away), what to eat (fruits, lots of vegetables, and other plants, as well as lots of fiber), and what to avoid (all processed and fast foods, and other foods that can spike the level of your blood sugar).

Thus, what you need to avoid AFib and other heart-related health complications is a combination of diets that guarantee that your heart and whole body are in good health. You'll be setting your tummy filled considerably, and the chances of getting hungry will become slimmer. AFib? That will be put into remission. If you're ready, let's take the tour.

Vegetables

Veggies are primarily the first to be considered in this chapter. Suppose you saw this coming, then good for you. And if you didn't, there's no need for you to feel bad. Even though the myriads of benefits that come with feeding on vegetables have been strongly emphasized and backed by much research, several people still don't see why this food should be given a priority. There are endless health benefits attached to eating veggies. And that includes the health of the heart because vegetables help in reducing inflammation and cutting visceral fats- two central stimulants of atrial fibrillation. Do you know the Mediterranean diet, the one based on natural plant-based foods? Yes, that's it- the one that has been revealed to reduce the risk of having AFib.

So, what quantity of vegetables should you be eating per day? Perhaps, the direction of that question should be changed: how many vegetables can you eat per day? Because as far as vegetables are concerned, there's almost no means of overdoing it. If you are complaining about not having enough to eat, vegetables are the way out.

You are not limited to a particular amount of vegetables; you are free to eat as much as you like. And the more you eat, the better your health and life become. So, eat broccoli as you've never done before. Chomp cauliflower like it's the only veggie in the universe. Please don't leave a carrot out; munch it. Your heart, without doubt, will be satisfied.

Here's the warning: vegetables like potatoes with a relatively high starch are not an option. Drenching vegetables with harmful oils such as processed sauces, cheeses, or ranch salad dressing are not the way out, either. The nearer to zero as you can get as far as eating harmful oils and starchy vegetables are concerned, the better for you.

However, in all their friendly, colorful, and tasty hodge-podge, raw or lightly cooked vegetables are the trick to weight reduction without feelings of hunger.

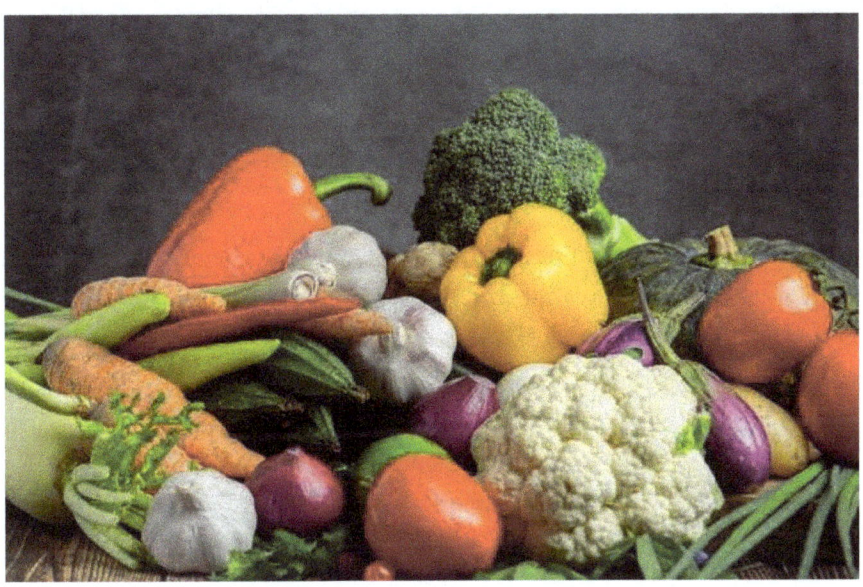

While you feed on vegetables, try as much as possible to optimize your nutrient. This is particularly important because tracking your nutrient intake will help you keep a relatively stable record of your weight over time while building improved data about your health and life. Unless you have been diagnosed with kidney failure, the more magnesium- and potassium-rich diets (that is, vegetables) you eat, the less your risk of having atrial fibrillation. The three most magnesium- and potassium-rich foods include beet greens, Swiss chard, and spinach. Other vegetables such as asparagus, broccoli, kale, Brussels sprouts, and cabbage are also rich in magnesium and potassium. Similarly, beans, fruits, nuts, and other seeds are rich in these nutrients.

To ensure that you are getting all the nutrients you need from these plant-based foods; you can use any smartphone app of your choice to track your micronutrients. A more straightforward approach is to consume as different colors as you can. You can take red, for instance, apples. Orange from Carrots. Yellow from Banana. Blue from blueberries. Green from spinach. Do you grab the concept? If you want to make it a bit simpler, you can make sure that all the rainbow colors are included in your combination. Boom! You'll quickly hit the nutrients you need this way.

Another thing that you need to know before you begin to compare your nutrients' level to that of another person is the freshness of what you are consuming. If a food, take a vegetable, for instance, had been out of the ground for a relatively long time, it will offer little or no nutrient at all to the body when it digests. So, what other options do you have? Well, there's another option. Have you thought of the flash-frozen organic frozen veggies? This option is a perfect one to consider.

Also, cooking your vegetables for a very long time will make them lose their nutrients and qualities that make them healthy choice of foods. Lightly cooked, tastily sautéed, raw, and broiled vegetables are all healthy choices. And, of course, if you are on meds, you will need to be extremely careful to avoid eating foods (vegetables) that will have adverse impacts on the drugs. You'll remember, for example, that warfarin thins the blood by blocking the passage of vitamin K. And since vegetables are very much high in this healthy vitamin, you will overwhelm the capacity of the blood thinner to stop the vitamin. If you're still interested in feeding on veggies, then you need to speak with your physician. He will probably prescribe another type of blood thinner that will not hinder the passage of vitamin K. If that option is not feasible, you can settle for a relatively steady amount of leafy greens and ask your doctor to adjust the dose of warfarin concerning your diet.

Telling some people to eat as many vegetables as possible per day isn't an ideal thing. More often than not, they are more pleased with a specific quantity. If you're looking for a more accurate measure of the number of vegetables that you should consume, then there's nothing more natural than your appetite. So let your appetite guide you; eat until you're satisfied. However, if all you still desire is a specific quantity, then do well to ensure that at least two-thirds to three-quarters of your meal is made up of vegetables. Instead of that, you can aim for five to six servings of veggies per day.

Fruits

This is another integral composition of the AFib diet. However, consumption of fruits essentially does not follow the same principle of "eat as much as you like" associated with vegetables. The reason is that some types of fruits can increase the level of your blood glucose drastically without offering similar rich complexity of minerals and vitamins that veggies may give.

All other things being equal, your best bet as far as fruits are concerned is berries, which have minimal effect on glucose and have been said to promote natural weight loss. Berries also contain fiber in high quantity. Two to three servings of fruits per day are a good goal, with berries constituting a more significant percentage. Bananas which you already know are very rich in potassium and magnesium are another healthy fruit option you should not do without. Would you mind not making the mistake of waiting until they become ripe before you eat them? If you want to get all the required nutrients out of them, eat them when they aren't too mature. Over-ripe bananas are known to spike the levels of blood glucose. Another healthy addition to your breakfast, lunch, and dinner is avocados. Avocados are generally rich in vitamin B, C, E, and K. They also contain niacin, folate, and riboflavin. Even tomatoes, exceptionally rich in fiber and potassium, can be a great option of fruit to add to your diet.

Whatever fruit you are eating, the best way to go about it is by ensuring that you eat as much of the whole fruit as possible and in its natural state. Unfortunately, rather than the natural fruit, many people prefer the processed counterparts. For example, they don't know a vast difference between orange and orange juice, which is just sugar water. Natural fruits help to retain the parts of the fruit that make the human body work harder to break it down and deliver nutrients that are often lost in the juice production process.

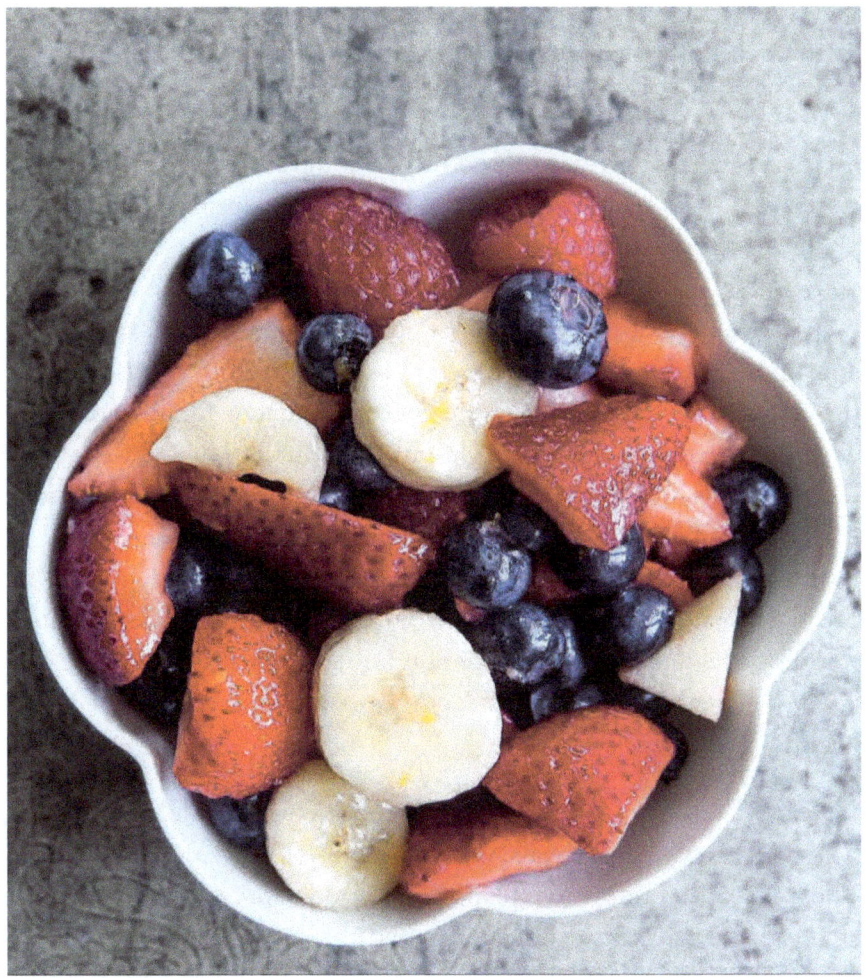

One particular fruit to which many individuals pay little or no attention to the side effects and continue to overeat is grapefruit. Research has shown that grapefruit can lengthen the QT interval on an EKG. You will be doing your health and whole life a lot of harm if you are on AFib medications that prolong QT interval such as sotalol, Multak (dronedarone), Tikosyn (dofetilide), or antidepressants; or amiodarone; or antibiotics. Suppose aren't sure if you are not sure if you should eat grapefruit, whether, in the natural form of the processed form, you should visit your physician for more clarification.

Grains are essentially harmful to most people suffering from atrial fibrillation. It is mainly a result of the substantial impacts of refined grains on excess weight gain and diabetes. The purpose of telling you this isn't so you can avoid taking grains. Instead, you can be meticulous in choosing the type of grain that you will eat. If you're considering eating grains, you should limit yourself to foods like brown rice and quinoa, which are yet to be pulverized into flour. Too many people believe that gluten-free flour and whole wheat, are healthy foods, but the reverse is true because these foods can spike your blood glucose level within a short period. Thus, bread isn't a healthy type of food, either. But if you can't do without eating bread, you should look out for the one that contains no flour. This flourless bread is made available in numbers in health food stores and mainstream supermarkets. You can grab one there to save your health.

Instead of eating veggies and veggies repeatedly, particularly in between heavy-veggie meals, you can choose to eat nuts and seeds. These are other innovative plant-based food sources that several studies have proved to contribute significantly to reducing AFib risk. For example, just a tiny helping of almonds, a few chia seeds, and a handful of pumpkin seeds can supply you with the much-required fiber, protein, magnesium, potassium, and other nutrients like the plant-derived fats, which have been revealed by studies to prevent the spike of blood glucose and promote healthy weight loss. In addition, dark chocolate and olive oil, both in very moderate quantities, are other plant-derived fat-containing diets that have been revealed to reduce the risk of having AFib. An added advantage of dark chocolates is that they are rich in AFib-suppressing nutrients magnesium and potassium.

Last but not least, consider legumes like lentils, chickpeas, beans, tamarinds, peanuts, and soybeans. These legumes are safe to consume and will considerably help in your fight against AFib.

Meat

The first time Devan was diagnosed with atrial fibrillation, he had just clocked 53 years. Every week after the first attack, he kept having episodes upon episodes, with some episodes lasting for as long as a whole day. It was a busy schedule for him because, at the time, he was running some computer software programs. But a miracle happened, just a year after he had suffered his first episode, his AFib episodes altogether ceased. How did he do it? Was he using any medication secretly, or had he undergone a procedure? Well, the truth is that he did none of those.

So, how? He had chosen to make a lot of optimized lifestyle changes. These helped him in the short run. But the significant and lasting changes came when he decided to make the right food choices food- he decided to settle for plant-based diets with wild meats accounting for a large percentage of his daily servings. After that, Devan related, he never had an episode of AFib even as he moved on to get involved in other life-challenging courses and tech startups.

"I knew what I was going through. Although my cardiologist seemed a little bit skeptical and unimpressed", Devan said. "But I knew I had found the perfect medication for my health in wild meats and vegetables; I knew if I could follow through, I would eventually be free."

Well, that was peculiar to Devan. But, of course, not everyone will have a similar story to tell. However, if you can make do with a 100 percent all-inclusive natural diet, meaning that a large part of it will be wild game, you may want to give it a try.

If carefully examined, Devan's food lifestyle can be compared with the eating habits of the Tsimane people. It is a tribe of hunter-gatherers of the lowlands of Bolivia who subsist on a diet of primary vegetables supplemented with fish and wild game. As a result, this tribe is said to have the lowest heart-related diseases and irregularities in the world. Almost not surprisingly, there are few or no cases of stroke or even atrial fibrillation among these people.

The reasons for the healthy heart and life associated with these people are not far-fetched. They do not eat sugar or processed foods. They live a slow-paced, technology-free, family-centered life. They spend about 7 hours each day foraging for food. Well, your guess can be pretty accurate. Of course, there might be some genetic factors responsible for their healthy life. Still, their level of commitment to maintaining this healthy life by eating more vegetables and wild meat cannot be underestimated.

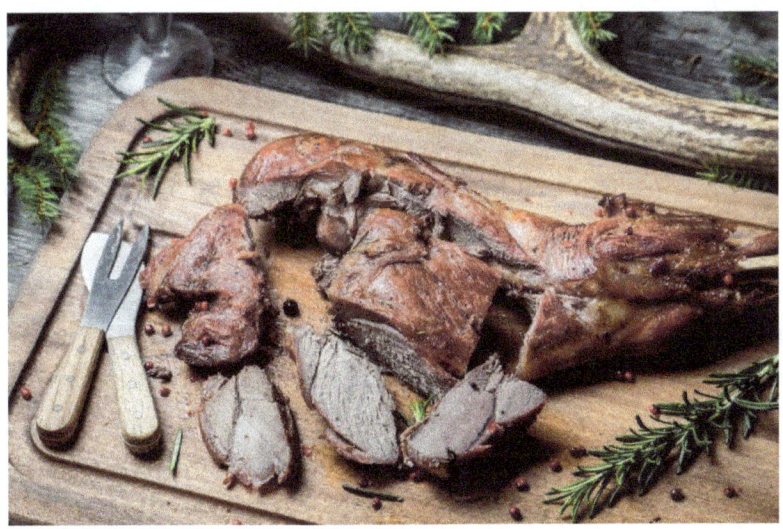

Irrespective of the reasons, studies of the Tsimane people further explain that meat isn't always unhealthy, as many people would argue. In comparison, some researchers have found a connection between meat consumption and the risk of heart infections, death caused by heart infections, and death in general. This is probably because most sampled people mainly were feeding on industrially processed meat alongside other unhealthy lifestyle habits. On the other hand, the meat that the Tsimane people eat does not come from animals packed in corrals, kept in a small-/medium-sized cages, slaughtered, packaged in nylon/plastic, and transported over hundreds of miles only to sit in a freezer in a grocery store. As such, it will be wrong to conclude that everyone can eat as much meat as they want just because some tribe of people consumes similar food substances without suffering any adverse health impacts. That's worth considering, especially when foods such as deli meats, bacon, and hotdogs have been revealed to contain chemicals known as carcinogens. Furthermore, these meats are not natural; they are densely processed.

Imitating the eating habits of the Tsimane people can be pretty tricky for some people. Even Devan acknowledged the fact that getting foods such as wild meats was a difficult task. He could only get the little he had because he had the connection and the means to access that source of food.

Well, there's another option, in this case, so you aren't out of luck. For you and several others who may not have access to wild game, fish can be your healthiest and most accessible source of animal protein. It is not just any type of fish, by the way, but wild fish that is rich in healthy doses of omega-3 fatty acids without any doe of PCBs and mercury. You can easily recall the type of fish that belong to this group using the acronym SMASH. This acronym stands for salmon, mackerel, anchovies, sardines, and herring. If steamed in an unhealthy way, these fish can also be dangerous to human health. Whatever nutrients you will be deriving from these fish will be destroyed when you choose to fry, batter, or drench them in unhealthy oils. Just like grains and vegetables, a fish offers the fullest nutritional benefits when it is lightly cooked, or let's say, when it still looks like a fish.

A research carried out on more than 5000 people showed that frequent fish consumers had a 31 percent reduced chance of suffering AFib episodes. While not every research has indicated that fish offers protection against AFib (and after several years of studies, there is no clear evidence of any AFib benefits derived from fish oil, either). Also, there's no evidence from these studies that SMASH fish steamed in healthy ways can increase your risk of atrial fibrillation.

Yet, it is necessary for you to recall that fish, just like meat, increases the secretion of TMAO. What this means is that there is that the connection between atrial fibrillation and fish consumption is nonlinear with very minimal befits but lots of harm. This is the reason you will likely see an equivalent of one or two savings of wild fish in large quantities week in week out in every AFib diet.

Why the equivalent? The culinary principles of persons from much distanced East Asian countries like Korea, China, and Japan, where very little meat is used to nourish vegetable dishes are quintessential for cooking good meat that is harmless to the heart. It shows that people living in these parts of the world choose to use meat the same way vegetables are used in the Western regions.

Rather than a large salmon steak served with a bit of quantity of asparagus by the side, think about a large plate of veggies coupled with a bit of toss of salmon. Even among people who choose to eat these Far East Asian diets, obesity is almost nonexistent. Studies have also shown that the risk of having AFib amongst those who cultivate this eating habit is ten times lower, unlike in the United States.

Fiber

You can't be hungry and say you are fighting against atrial fibrillation. That's a double whammy. So, you'll likely need something to keep you full. Well, the best option you can have is fiber. That's because fiber (the part of plant-based diets that can't be broken down during the process of digestion) increases the urge of feeling full by as much as 38 percent, according to a review of forty-four published research by the researchers of the University of Minnesota. The outcome of this is a massive decrease in the intake of calories. The equation is relatively easy to grasp: the more fiber you eat, the lower your weight. And the lower your weight, the lower the amount of visceral fat you carry about. And the lower the amount of visceral fat in your body, the lower the risk of developing AFib. In addition, in research conducted by the University of Helsinki, fiber was found to be effective in preventing blood glucose spikes.

So, in what type of foods are you likely to find the highest amount of fiber? Plants of all kinds (you should have now known that meat doesn't contain fiber at all). Diets such as berries, vegetables, beans, lentils, chia seeds, and peas are all intelligent and healthy sources of fiber. If you want to add more fiber, say for desserts, you can make do with healthy dark chocolate, which contains cocoa with little or no added sugar.

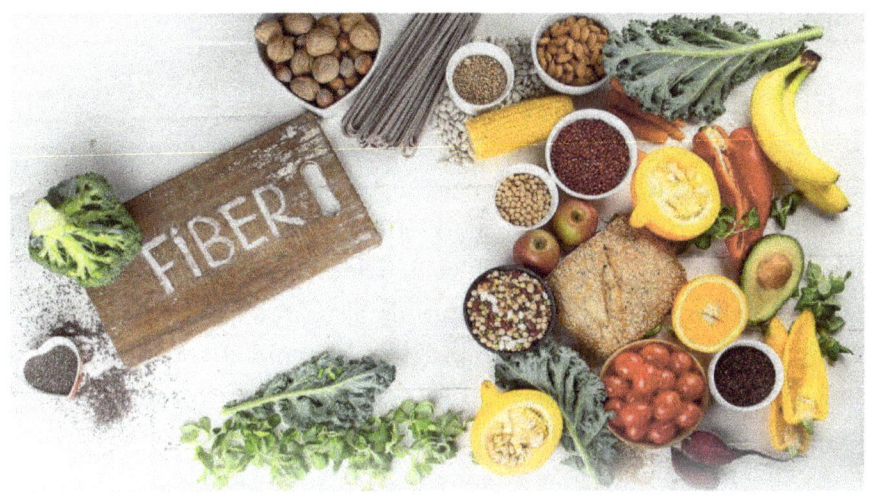

By eating more of these diets, you are increasingly reducing your vulnerability to atrial fibrillation. Several years of research back it. Researchers have discovered a statistical trend of about 36 percent reduced risk of AFib among people who feed on large quantities of fiber. The study was based on a group of people with the highest consumption of about 27 grams of fiber per day, and that's way below the 100 to 150 measure of fiber that the contemporary-time hunter-gathering people and our Paleolithic ancestors consumed. You can set this goal for yourself and aim at accomplishing it. You also have the opportunity to hit 100 grams of fiber without necessarily taking fiber supplements if you eat veggie-dense foods in large amounts.

Nuts and Seeds

If you were a voracious consumer of nuts as far back as eighty years ago, you would probably have been tagged a "nutty" by several people. Since 1960, for instance, the Blue Diamond's campaign labeled "a can per day, that's all we demand" has incredibly increased the consumption of almonds by tenfold. Yet, despite that, many people whose aim was to lose weight avoided nuts because they contain many fats and calories, even as further research demonstrated that not all calories and fats are equal.

Across the the United States, consumption of almonds has considerably replaced peanuts over the years. Although this trend has gained popularity in every part of the country, several other nuts are incredibly rich in nutrients that are neglected. Think about it, nuts such as macadamias, cashew, Brazil nuts, walnuts, hazelnuts, pecans, and several others share the same nutritional values as almonds. And yes, that same nutritional value is present in that decorated legume, always taking the appearance of a nut: peanut.

Do you want to lose weight in the next couple of months? Why not give nuts a try? Nuts play a very incredible role in weight loss. All of those proteins, fats, and fiber make you filled up. So you can trust nuts to boost your metabolism. A study conducted to validate the nutritional status of almonds, for instance, showed that people who included almonds in their daily servings were able to lose as much as 65 percent of their weight compared to their non-almond-eating counterparts. While that impact seems a bit inconclusive concerning the observations of other studies, the total of the evidence suggests that nuts of all kinds either assist in weight loss or, at the very least, have no role to play in weight gain. It means that the consumption of nuts, in general, helps you to add healthy fats and protein without the adverse health effects that come with excess meat consumption.

That's a conclusion that is backed by another research-based fact about nuts: eating nuts reduces your risk of suffering any heart as well as atrial fibrillation.

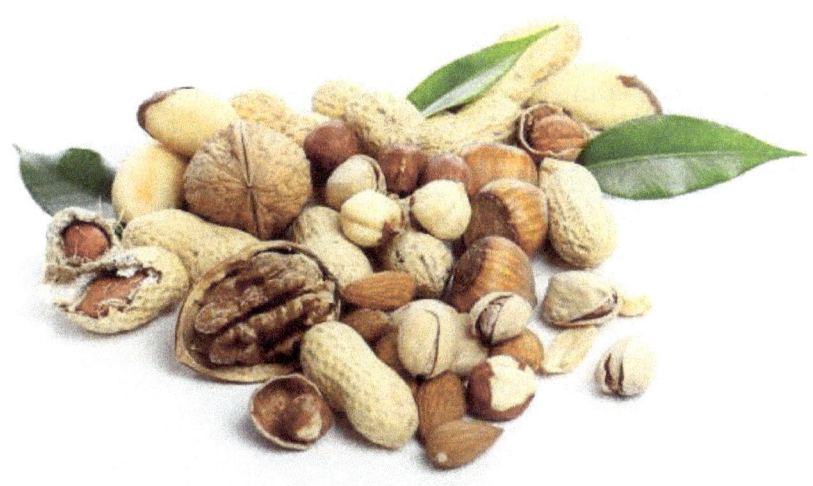

However, there are certain things that you should put into consideration before eating nuts. For instance, the gussied-up types of nuts that have become so common in recent years should be avoided. These versions often contain a high amount of sugar, salt, and preservatives that hinder positive health benefits. If at all you want to add some flavor to these treats, you can do that in the closet of your home with a pinch of chili, garlic, or onion powder, or a squirt of hot sauce and a dash of lemon juice.

You might be wondering why things you shouldn't even consider eating are yet to be discussed in this chapter, and that notion might have been geared in your mind because as far as diets are concerned, what comes first are the warnings and prohibitions. However, the reverse is the case here. A look at what you should eat before you think about what you shouldn't eat is crucial. By adhering strictly to the number of duets that have been provided so far, you will notice a significant reduction in your consumption of those things you shouldn't eat. It will get to a point those things will "smell foul" to you. And that's the excellent news: avoiding diets that make you more vulnerable to developing atrial fibrillation.

Let's take a turn at this juncture and look at those things you need to avoid.

Eliminate Processed Foods

Over the years, there have been increasing marketers whose first and foremost goal is to spur consumers to eat by taking the conventional means of branding and tagging all foods "healthy." What they do is stack these foods in muted brown or green boxes, then go ahead to proclaim their "natural" sweetness and "organic" credentials during an advertisement.

You can say it; marketing is a captivating adventure. Also, there's nothing wrong with trying to persuade a person that instead of a Product X, you should choose to spend your money on a Product Y. However, the big problem with these marketers' agents is that they are just trying to shift your attention from a particular brand. Their ultimate goal is to give you a highly different pattern of food consumption.

Here's the fact that you should be well aware of: packaged foods, irrespective of how fancy and pleasant marketers and producers present them, are processed foods. In addition, in the process of improving their life span, many chemicals and preservatives are used in making them. Thus, little does it matter that their producers and marketers proclaim their healthiness during adverts. A label or tag does not make food healthy.

So, how do you know that food is processed? It's pretty easy to determine. Processed foods are usually very different from the natural substances they were made of and are often prepared or steamed up with a large amount of salt and sugar.

You don't need to take a walk too far before you discover that most Americans get a considerable amount of sodium in their foods, and the reason for that is not because they are too free with the salt shaker; instead, it owes mainly to the fact that more often than not, processed foods are swimming in salt. As you grow older, the amount of salt you need to stay healthy becomes less. Studies have demonstrated that individuals above the age of fifty need less than one gram of sodium per day compared to younger individuals. More so, salt is added to many of the common foods that you purchase for texture, taste, and as a preservative. You shouldn't be surprised at this point to learn that excess salt in your nutrition is a potential risk for developing atrial fibrillation. Hence, the safest option would be to reduce or even eliminate prepared, packaged, or processed foods.

Here's the shocker. There are some food products, available in their countless figures, that don't even attempt to appear healthy. You know them too well: plastic-packaged cookies and cakes, soft drinks, freezer meals, and several others. It is a front to human decency and good sense to refer to these products as "foods." Instead, what could be more suitable is "Frankenfoods" or "food-like products," as they have little or no nutritional value attached.

From bottled sauces to boxed cereals to canned soups, processed foods are generally not suitable for anyone and are incredibly detrimental to the health of those who want to decrease their risk of AFib.

The same applies to fast foods. There's little, and that's if there's anything at all, that can be gotten from a drive-through that can even possibly be referred to as "healthy," let alone be considered harmless to eat without raising the risk of atrial fibrillation. These foods are designed to be "highly palatable" with heavy doses of sodium that increase fluid retention and blood pressure, a lot of sugar that spike blood glucose, plenty of unhealthy oils that destroy your cholesterol numbers, and several highly processed and industrially produced animal-based proteins that stimulate TMAO production.

Recently, many fast-food restaurants have begun gearing towards plant-based proteins made to look and taste very similar to animal protein. While there might have been many benefits alluded to these experiments in new food samples, especially in terms of the environmental impacts and moral implications of meat consumption, these are goods created in laboratories. These laboratory-created duets are densely processed, and since they have been designed to imitate animal proteins, they may come with many of the same potential health problems. Studies carried out foster our understanding of what those problems are; however, it's essential not to assume that "plant-based" means "eat as much as you like." These diets are not veggies.

There's another highly processed and fast food that only a few people know is a processed food, and it's a principal constituent of many people's nutrition. It's not so obvious, though. So, unless you are taking a walk around the market with one eye opened and intensely concentrated on foods to avoid just because they don't look like the natural ingredients from which they were made, you would probably make the mistake of purchasing them. Do you know the part of the market where you will most likely come across these foods? It is the bakery.

Loaves of bread are largely processed foods. They are usually jam-packed with many ingredients aimed at molding and staling for a relatively long period. And despite this, many people, particularly those whose elementary school teacher did well to teach them that cereals and loaves of bread form the central base of the food pyramid, have now regarded bread as an integral part of a healthy balanced diet. The belief that bread is a portion of healthy food is further reiterated by the Judeo-Christian idea of "daily bread," which depicts that rather than what one wants, bread is what one needs. But taking a closer look at this idea, based on the research that scholars and experts have made, that "daily" as used in this prayer means "super substantial," you will see that the word is more of transcendent needs than about literal food. You don't need to travel back in time to know that the loaves of bread commonly available in most supermarkets today are often made with processed flour and are dissimilar to the bread eaten in Biblical periods.

Most modern loaves of bread are a twofold blow, for real. First, they are processed, but the processing also converts the essential ingredients into something significantly wrong for people with AFib: sugar.

Do Away With Blood Sugar Spikes

Joe had a well-paying job. He was working as a system engineer in a big tech company. You could tell that he was satisfied with the job and the atmosphere surrounding the job. He was irrevocably committed to his career. He soon developed a lot of heart complications. As a result, he suffered from high blood pressure, excess weight gain, diabetes, and of course, atrial fibrillation. It didn't take too long for Joe to find out that carbohydrates, mainly any food containing added sugar or flour, are great stimulants responsible for dramatic blood sugar spikes.

Vegetables that contain little or no amount of starch cannot cause a spike in blood glucose levels. Fruits are another safe option, that's if you choose to consume moderately. You will be doing your health a lot of harm if you eat overripe or tropical fruits. If you want to keep your blood sugar under control, berries are the safest option. Legumes are low glycemic, too. However, when grains are ground into a fine powder, they are easily converted into sugar in the body.

After a lot of research and a critical look at the available options, the "avoid sugar like the plague" option seemed to Joe the suitable alternative to choose. He knew that if he was going to get out of the situation he was in, he had to avoid blood sugar spikes. Frankly, the principles of ketogenic diets aren't a bad starting point for fighting atrial fibrillation, as a low-glycemic food is essential to those for whom a spike in blood sugar can be both a trigger and substrate cause of the arrhythmia.

Joe, who wanted to go back to his everyday healthy life, wasn't interested in the "mild keto" approach many people try by attempting to limit carbs. So, he purchased a ketone meter, which examines the chemicals produced by the liver when the body lacks sufficient insulin to convert sugar into energy, and ensure that day after day, he reached this level of "ketosis," which is characterized by the capacity of the body to burn fat for energy as a result of lack of carbohydrates. Then, he proceeded to graph the outcome with the kind of precision that befits his engineering background. Indeed, it was a beauty to behold.

Although some researchers have found some connections between atrial fibrillation and low-carb foods, it has also been discovered that people who eat foods in very unhealthy ways after quitting carbs are the most susceptible to AFib.

With a large number of veggies and moderate consumption of berries, alongside healthy fats, Joe was able to put his excess weight, diabetes, hypertension, and other health complications into remission within one month. However, he later found out that his "true keto" food robbed him of the magnesium and potassium needed to combat his AFib. He also discovered that excess meat pushed him out of ketosis. It makes a lot of sense since the extra protein in most of the foods you consume can be easily converted to sugar by the body.

He did increase his consumption of low-glycemic magnesium- and potassium-rich veggies and reduce the amount of meat. And just with that, he was fine. His health complications were nowhere to be found, and the number of drugs he takes every day reduced to zero.

CHAPTER TWO:

MAKING IT WORK FOR YOU

Centenarians are mainly known to live in good health until nature calls, their younger counterparts seldom have that privilege. And there's a lot of sense in this. To reach an advanced age, you must have had all your cards played right.

Despite this fact, more than a quarter of centenarians living in the United States have AFib. In Denmark and Spain, for instance, it's about one in every five.

But there are some regions in the world where the rate is much lower. One of such regions is the village of Bapan, which borders across the Panyang River in Southern China. The rate of atrial fibrillation amongst centenarians in this part of the world is lower than one out of twenty.

The Village of Bapan is a region in China that has long been known for its significant number of people who live beyond one hundred. And almost all of these individuals mark their centenary age in good health. Some of them even work at this age. So it's pretty surprising.

You're probably asking yourself at this moment if these people could have inherited some sorts of genes that make them live for that long. Maybe. However, research has revealed that the inhabitants of this village have a few markers that indicate increased risks of various kinds of chronic diseases.

How? The principles of Longevity Village can be broken down into four significant rules that can help you live a better and healthier life.

- Eat good food
- Rule your mindset
- Never be sedentary
- Build yourself a place in a healthy society
- Find a rhythm

Bobby was in his early forties when he suffered his first episode of atrial fibrillation. That was as far back as the early 2000s; he was in his mid-fifties at the time. At that particular time when it happened, Bobby wasn't doing anything that could have triggered an episode of atrial fibrillation.

"I was just there, just meditating. Nothing more", said Bobby, a project supervisor in a city university. "I was just there, calm and quiet, in the middle of an array of thoughts going through my mind. And just suddenly, I felt my heart pounding away rapidly like a spark between the negative ends of two cables. But this time, the spark continued and kept going on and on and on. It was like my heart was going to come out of my chest. So awkward".

Meditation has been verified as one of the Eastern-informed approaches for reducing the risk of atrial fibrillation. What this means is that Bobby's experience was quite unusual. So it's possible, in fact, very probable, that meditation didn't play a role in the AFib attack that Bobby had. It just occurred to me what he was doing at the moment when all of the other underlying factors that were immensely contributing to his condition joined forces together to create an arrhythmia.

Years after that initial frightening attack, Bobby had put in a lot of effort to find out the substrate causes and triggers of his AFib. Over time, he came up with the principle that "pursuing every possible trigger" can solve the problem. But that principle had diminishing returns attached to it. Thus, he needed another approach, an all-inclusive one at that.

And that begins with food. Not just any sort of food, but excellent and nutritious food. Food that supplies the body with the necessary nutrients needed to keep it healthy and active. Also, it must be food that you want to eat. You can't just pack a load of foods without being ready to eat them.

"I tell others the good news. The news that they need to eat better and try to eat good food. The news that clean food without junk is the ultimate way out", he said. "I've been committed to all of that, as well."

For Bobby, that means a lot of organic paleo and plant-based foods, including fresh veggies, in addition to some supplementations for nutrients needed by his body, and for some other not-so-obvious reasons, elements such as magnesium, potassium, and vitamin D.

For instance, as far as potassium is concerned, Bobby gets almost everything that he needs from food. However, you'll still find him with a bottle of potassium chloride tablets because there can be an urgent need for the supplement at any time. "So if I had gone through a lot of stress like if I had been out in the yard throughout the day, perhaps during summer, and had I had no strength to get some foodstuff, I'll just settle for a dose."

Staying committed to eating good food for as long as you live can be quite a challenging task for many individuals, especially in this current time where you are bombarded with several options to stray away from diets that help keep your heart in rhythm. You can't afford to do that. If you want to push atrial fibrillation into total remission, you must be irrevocably committed to eating good foods.

Rule Your Mindset

What do most AFib patients stand to lose when they are diagnosed with the disease? First, of course, many people would say it is their normal heart rhythm. But that is not always the case. Second, people seem to pay less attention to the fact that atrial fibrillation robs you of your strength and a positive mindset. Third, it reduces the time and opportunities you have to participate in the things you love actively.

More often than not, atrial fibrillation comes with despondency and hopelessness. In addition, researchers have revealed that people diagnosed with AFib often have symptoms of depression and that these symptoms have the potential of exacerbating their AFib symptoms, thereby resulting in a devastating vicious cycle.

Bella Croft could perhaps better understand this subject. She was the sole proprietor of an art gallery located at the center of the city. If you were looking for a place to behold the artistic beauties of not just the American territories, but also the world at large, her gallery was the right place to visit. She was fifty at the time, and you could say she was on top of her game.

"I was always on the move," she explained, she was almost everywhere at the same time, traveling from one country to another, and "always on airplanes."

"Then it happened. I had just returned from a trip that day and was resting on the sofa, checking and going through my emails, when suddenly, my heart skipped a beat and began racing. I couldn't do anything. So I just lay right there on the sofa while my husband came running towards me with blood pressure cuff".

"It wasn't even cold weather at the time. My husband reported having noticed my right leg become as white as snow. Even in the warm weather, I felt cold, and my sight was kind of blurry. The doctor I had met at the emergency room told me I had had blood clots and would have suffered a stroke from a heart condition called atrial fibrillation, which I had never come across before".

And like many doctors would do, Bella's doctor told her that the best option for fighting against AFib was using meds including blood thinners and beta-blockers, the former of which made her suffer bruises all over. "It was unpleasant, "she remembered.

And even with the meds, Bella didn't notice any significant improvement in her condition. "It takes a huge toll on your physical health," she said. "If you suffer from paroxysmal atrial fibrillation when it's over with you after the first episode, you feel so down, and all you will want to do at that point is to sleep. You're completely wiped out. So, it takes a toll on your physical well-being. And your emotional well-being, too. You're just frightened thinking about when another episode is going to show up again. The fear of telling your family you can't plan that event again or even go out with them grips you".

Just as Bella was beginning to recognize that her life was drawing nearer to a conclusive end, she had a moment of fortune. She came across an article on ablation procedure, and just in few weeks, she was wearing a brown gown.

"Afterwards, I became free from AFib," she said, "and I've always been free since then."

While Bella's ablation procedure helped her put atrial fibrillation into remission, it took total devotion to lifestyle optimization to keep it off. And it's possible that the endless hope that characterized her life before the episode, and the optimism gathered after her ablation procedure, were great contributing factors, as well.

Hope isn't something you can decide to turn on and later turn off again. However, it is something you can improve upon if you discipline yourself.

Thus, if you want to push your AFib into complete remission and have it stay off, an optimistic mindset is indispensable. So, build that mindset.

Don't be Sedentary

It was now some decades later after he had suffered his first episode of atrial fibrillation, Bobby was still committed to his healthy feeding habits, as well as other lifestyle optimizations, and you could see that he was happy, healthy, and his heart was in perfect rhythm.

He was still given regular medication, but that didn't stop his veggies. Neither did it stop his steady and consistent exercise.

That last part could not be overlooked. Of course, you are aware that plenty of exercises are an integral part of lifestyle optimization. One thing that you might not have a clear understanding of yet is how easy this approach is. You can make it a lot easier for you by substituting the concept of "exercise" with the word "motion." This way, you ease yourself of the "burden" many people perceive regular exercise as.

- Rigorous exercise

This is the type that makes you breathe heavily and sweat profusely, is quite essential. But you do not necessarily need such exercise in large amounts. You might recall from the previous chapter where lifestyle optimizations were analyzed that five to ten minutes of intense vigorous exercise is sufficient. And too much rigorous exercise (engaging in competitive endurance sports/activities) can induce an AFib attack.

So, what type of exercise do you need? All that is required by your body is the sort of exercise that gives it a good dose of continuous, low-level physical stress. It is the type that will make you break a sweat and breathe a little bit harder but doesn't gets your clothes soaked with sweat or leave you gasping for air, thereby raising the rate of your heartbeat. To be more explicit, this is the type of exercise you need by simply being in motion.

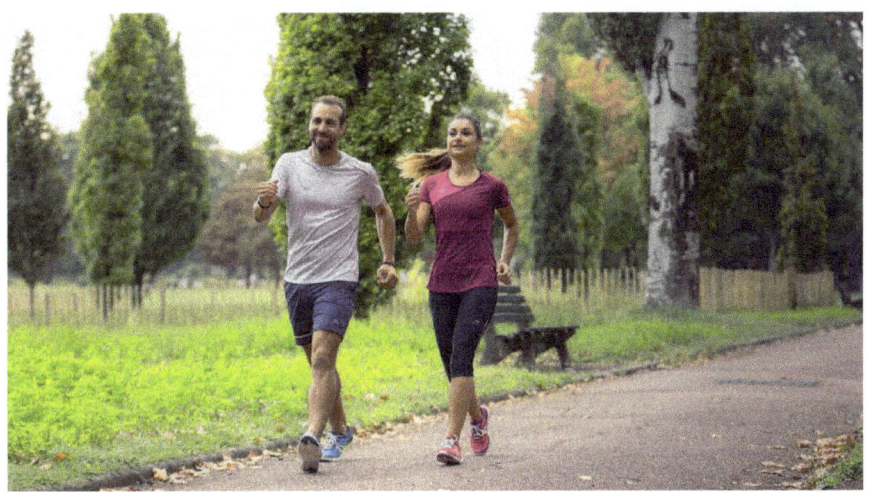

If your job means working in an office building, for instance, staying in motion means refusing to use the elevator and daily commitment to using the stairs instead. You can devise other healthy means such as setting up a walking group at lunchtime or arranging a small piece of exercise pedals beneath your desk; for those who want to keep moving even while at work, a standing treadmill desk can be beneficial. Without doubt, it will take a relatively long time to get used to working while walking, but studies have indicated that individuals who use standing treadmill desks are not less productive compared to their sitting counterparts; they are just healthier.

If you are a great fan of TV programs, or you're retired and, for that reason, are often sedentary, you can change your "daily watch" habits into something that's of more significant meaning. How do you go about that? Machines such as elliptical machines, exercise bikes, and treadmills can give you a conscience-free way of watching your programs. This way, you will be able to transform an activity that's quite unhealthy into something that is not just beneficial to your physical appearance but the health of your body in general.

If you are perhaps an endurance athlete, it is vital that you are smart about your rate of exercise, particularly if you've had your AFib ablated at one point before. Undergoing excess stress can increase your risk of atrial fibrillation. The long-term adverse effects of continuous rigorous exercise can cause electrical and structural changes in the heat that can incite atrial fibrillation. The truth is that almost anyone is vulnerable to AFib if their body is subjected to too much stress. There have been many cases of very young and very healthy adults who have developed AFib due to their involvement in a motor vehicle accident, or a massive infection, or surgery. Pushing yourself to do beyond what you have been trained to do can also make you vulnerable to suffering AFib.

The reason you need to stay in motion is beyond putting AFib into remission; it borders around engaging in exercise even unintentionally to keep the disease off totally. Don't be sedentary.

Build Yourself a Place in a Healthy Society

You all remember Debbie? After undergoing an ablation procedure, she had to make plans with her immediate society (her family) to help her keep the disease at bay forever. It means that if you ever want to make it work for you, you will need the help of the people around you. You can't possibly do it alone. Therefore, you will need your family to understand the goal and what it will take for you to achieve it. Your family can turn out to be the only society you need if the members are willing and ready to actively help you and even make sacrifices to assist you in reaching your goal of a better and healthier life.

However, not everyone shares the same luck as Debbie. And it's not difficult at all to find people who have AFIB who want to eat better and healthier but whose family members gather around pizza, hamburger, or fried chicken each time dinner is set. There are many stories of husbands who are very much aware of the dire need of their wives to get enough exercise to keep their hearts in rhythm, but would never rise to join them in the process. If you find yourself in such a situation, it isn't that you have the wrong family; it's just that you are yet to find the perfect healthy society to help you achieve your goal of fighting against AFib. A fight against AFib that will make you sad is not worth it, so you'll need to find your perfect environment somewhere else.

Your colleagues and friends are other great options. However, this option might as well not often turn out as positive as you desire. For example, friends and colleagues might love to get together late at night to have a few drinks. At this point, you know that you are making yourself vulnerable to two underlying factors that can cause AFib. Sometimes, you might get invited to lunch in a restaurant where the only healthy option available on the menu is a bottle of water.

What do you do now that all options seem to be exhausted? Why not think outside the box? There are many forums and networks of people worldwide who know what it takes to fight against atrial fibrillation. In your community, in your state, in your country, even with the aid of the internet, you can find some of these forums and networks in large numbers. And not only is it easy to come across these groups of fellow AFib fighters, but you can also find a network of people who share similar AFib experiences as you.

While the first and foremost aim of whatever group you get yourself engaged in should help you kick out AFib completely, such groups don't need to be AFib concerted. It could be a religious study group, a softball team, or a knitting society. The only thing that you need is the feeling of comfort and daily devotion to maintaining a lifestyle that respects and supports your intention of pushing AFib into complete remission.

Find a Rhythm

Are you looking for a perfect metaphor for life? Then, AFib is. When your life is suddenly out of rhythm, it's almost often a piece of evidence that some other parts of your body are out of rhythm, as well. That can be medications, sleep, stress, exercise, metabolism, or any other underlying causes discussed in the first part. And more often than not, it is a collection of imbalances.

Once you can find a balance through lifestyle optimization, the goal is to maintain it. And the best way to do that is by taking a critical look at the first law of motion propounded by Sir Isaac Newton. You'll discover that this law isn't just a fundamental principle of mechanics; it's an essential lesson for maintaining a healthy life.

Do you remember that law? You were probably taught in the first or second year in middle school. OK, you don't need to fret if you don't remember. So let me help you out. The first law of Sir Isaac Newton states that objects at rest will remain at rest, while things in motion will stay in motion unless acted upon by an external force.

Humans generally aren't different from comic dust; better still, meteoroids coming and going through space. But, once we begin to move and gain a little momentum behind us, there's every tendency that we become committed to that pace. The problem is that the lessons we've kept ourselves committed to for as long as we've been living are the paths that have led us to atrial fibrillation in the first place. Worse still, even if we devote ourselves to life changes and follow good habits, the world has at its disposal external forces aiming at pushing us off course.

In the midst of all this, how do you keep monitoring your biomarkers, keeping a continuous process of lifestyle optimization, and keeping track of your wellness?

If your physician, tells you that your body requires 30 minutes of moderate work-out per day, you can go for 60 or even more on weekends when you have ample time at your disposal. If, by tracking your wellness, you discover that your heart is most likely to be in rhythm when you meditate in the evening, you should engage in that stress-easing exercise in the morning, as well. If your episodes of atrial fibrillation stay at a relatively low ebb even when your biomarkers are a bit down or high, continue making attempts to bring those figures into a better and healthier range.

Don't wait until things become complicated before you begin to make these life-transforming decisions. Instead, make them while the times are good when everything looks okay and when it's been so long, you last suffered an episode of AFib that you seem to forget if you were once at risk. This way, when things become more and more complicated, you'll have the momentum you need to confront the odds that come your way without having to risk your health and life.

That was one of the principles that helped Bobby stay focused even after the ablation procedure. He was able to recognize the power of the procedure after that. For almost a decade after being diagnosed with AFib, he addressed it with lifestyle optimization alone and didn't perceive a procedure as an option. "If I had been told I would later settle for ablation, I would have laughed it off," he related. "Then, I got the strength, the energy to make that decision as time drew nearer. And believe me, it was worth it because then, I had mastered my atrial fibrillation ".

Like Bobby, many people can end their AFib if they are willing and ready to embrace the procedure and the optimizations. So, therefore, whether it's having an ablation, or running an extra mile each week, or spending more time tracking your numbers, or focusing on a few more biomarkers, or doing anything you can do to keep your heart in rhythm and keep your life in balance even when AFib tries to throw odds at you, don't give up; do it.

Summarized below are the Bapan lessons in more relatable format. The beauty of doing this is to enable you to have a quick reminder of these lessons so as to stay committed to them as you go out and come in every day.

- Eat Good Food
- Follow a diet that helps you to lose weight considerably. Also, you must try as much as possible to maintain a healthy weight for a long time without any fluctuations.
- If the diet you are taking isn't addressing your arrhythmia and weight, you should opt for the AFib diet.
- Do away with processed and fast foods completely
- Rule Your Mindset
- Replace pessimistic beliefs with optimistic alternatives.
- Have a positive and healthy view about the future. Don't stress your mental health with vain imaginations.
- Start each day with activities that enhance positivity
- Don't Be Sedentary
- Try as much as possible to stay in motion for at least half of your working hours.
- Irrespective of where you are starting from, incorporate more motion and productive exercise into your life as you age.

- Take active part in vigorous exercise for at least few minutes, few times every day.
- Build Yourself A Place in a Healthy Society
- Demand the assistance of families and friend to help you achieve your goal.
- Don't get cross with unsupportive individuals. If they aren't contributing positively to your health and life, you should say good-bye. If they are indispensable in your life, just recognize that they aren't in the best position to help at that moment.
- Seek alternative support groups in your community, state, country, and even via online means.
- Find a Rhythm
- Begin with as much momentum as possible.
- Don't settle for less. Go far above the minimum.
- Build a routine in correlation to your AFib-fighting lifestyle.

CHAPTER THREE:

AFIB IS NOT YOUR END; IT IS ONLY THE BEGINNING OF A BETTER AND HEALTHIER LIFE

Maybe it might look inappropriate or even awkward to congratulate people on being diagnosed with AFib. After all, this is a medical condition that changes many people's lives for the worse, subjects them to some devastatingly wrong medications, and drives them down a steep road to more and more health complications. A third is likely to suffer from stroke. Even those who live for a considerably long time will have an increased risk of dementia. Worst still, for as many as, would adopt them; conventional treatments won't lead to a significantly better and healthier long-term quality of life.

However, you deserve being congratulated if you've been diagnosed with atrial fibrillation.

If you have found out that you have an increased risk of developing AFib, you also deserve a congratulation.

If you have a friend, relative, or loved one suffering from atrial fibrillation and you intend to give them the hope of better and improved life, you too deserve being congratulated.

If you've been diagnosed with atrial fibrillation, and you're just tired about everything, well, I owe you congratulations.

You know why?

Because there's hope as long as you are alive, and there's a solution, a path. Many people have walked this path, and many people are just getting to know about it now. It is a path to a better and healthier life- not just healthier than life is currently, but potentially more beneficial than life has ever been.

The pounding, and the breathlessness, and the throbbing, and the exhaustion, and the fear that characterize atrial fibrillation are signs that what you need to do is making significant lifestyle changes that will improve your overall health. They are the body's caveat sirens. Something has likely gone wrong somewhere, and many things will go wrong if you decide to do nothing to address the situation. Therefore, it is the perfect time to control the things that triggered those sirens on and the moment to make the decisions that are capable of turning those sirens off and keeping them off for as long as you live.

Indeed, it's safer never to have had to make those decisions in the first instance, but the deed has been done. Your past is your past. And your today is your today. All you have now is to correct those wrongs. Your future is your future, and between your past and your future, the future indeed can be brighter.

And for that reason, congratulations. That is your big moment.

As you have found out, the atrial fibrillation cure isn't a set of principles. Instead, it's a process of decisions, goals, evaluations, and reassessment. It's a lifetime devotion to health, fulfillment, and happiness. However, one fact should not be underestimated. It is a process based on myriads of promising research, including a brilliant study by electrophysiologist Dr. Prash Sanders.

Dr. Sanders specializes in the area of cardiac ablation at the University of Adelaide in Australia. It has a public access health system with generally good results across the country. Nevertheless, like any other public system, it has demerits, as well. At the period when the EP started his practice, one of such demerits was that cardiac ablation was covered irregularly in various territories and states. Ironically, this resulted from the fact that nothing was left in the body after the completion of the procedure. And for several years in Australia, reimbursement was compulsory for many implantable heart tools, including pacemakers, stents, and defibrillators (not used for ablation in this case). The outcome was a lengthy list of people waiting to receive ablation.

"As drugs were no longer helping the situations of these patients, I had nothing more at my disposal to offer them as they waited for almost a year for their ablation procedure," the EP explained.

During the long wait, the EP advised these patients to attempt a lifestyle optimization approach. This multidisciplinary strategy also has, as an integral part of it, the weight-loss program. And finding this as an opportunity to pool data, the doctor followed them up closely. "I was amazed at what I saw. What I noticed was that as these patients lost weight, there was a significant reduction in AFib symptoms", he said.

This spurred the Journal of the American College of Cardiology to mount further research into the subject. The good news is that the outcome of the study correlated with the EP's findings. Tremendously, over five years, about 46 percent of people who were able to shed a significant percentage of their weight (an average of 35 pounds) put their AFib into remission up to the point that they no longer required medications or an ablation.

However, this category of people didn't just benefit from the highly reduced rate of atrial fibrillation. After all, when people lose weight, their health improves gradually in other areas, too. For example, among those suffering from hypertension, systolic blood pressure reduced by 18 points on average; that relatively notes than two times the reduction achieved by the average blood pressure drug. In addition, inflammation, measured using C-reactive protein, dropped by 76 percent; that's essentially a helpful finding because inflammation of the heart is one of the major underlying causes of scarring or fibrosis, which eventually leads to atrial fibrillation.

LDL cholesterol which increases the risk of having heart diseases, dropped to as low as 16 percent. Triglyceride levels, which have been associated with AFib, strikes, and heart attack, were reduced by 31 percent. There was also a tremendous improvement of 18 percent in the thickness and dilation of their heat as measured using an echocardiogram. In a more relatable term, their hearts changed into much better and healthier-functioning organs.

Also, in what was perceived to be the best evidence to show that attempts made at addressing the problems that lead to AFib, will positively affect other diseases, there was a vast 88 percent of people in the group who had their diabetes pushed into complete remission, getting the level of their hemoglobin A1C back to its normal range through weight loss.

Not surprisingly, there was also an average of 200 percent improvement in the well-being of the patients in this group. It was a self-reported feeling and can be said to have been due to their devotion to life-transforming decisions. It is no new news that no antidepressants in the world have achieved so much impact as this.

That's just a focus on weight loss. If you combine these impacts with the improvements that come from monitoring and tracking biomarkers, other optimized lifestyle changes such as better sleep and reduced stress, the life-transforming power of an ablation procedure (for those who need it), a decrease in the dependency on medications, and a lifetime devotion to tracking your wellness, the outcome isn't just better and improved health; it could be a cure for a lifetime.

Conclusion – Part 3

A Life after AFib

You sure have learned a lot from every page of this book. You've learned about the stories of others. There was Maria who confronted her condition by changing her work. Debbie also took to the procedure of ablation but had to resort to lifestyle optimization to put the disease into total remission.

In addition, there were cases of Fagin, Shaw, Gina, Flora, and several others who committed themselves to transformational life decisions that helped them win in the end. And there were many others, too, who became victims of atrial fibrillation from different backgrounds and as a result of various underlying factors but were desperately in search of a solution to make sure that this horrible condition didn't define whom they turned out to be.

Now is the time you will decide what story you will be telling in the next few months or years. Are you ready to reverse, and if possible, eliminate atrial fibrosis and atrial fibrillation from developing? Will you be irrevocably committed to biomarker monitoring? What about lifestyle optimization? Are you willing to follow the processes thoroughly until you begin to see some positive changes? Will you begin to take the bold steps needed to avoid taking unnecessary meds? What about tracking your wellness? Are you willing and ready to monitor your sleep, food, medications, exercise, stress, blood pressure, amongst others, to ensure improvements don't retract as the years pass by?

If you're willing and ready to embark on this life-changing adventure, then there's an assurance your big dream will very soon become a reality. The life ahead is full of bliss.

So, never stop the beats. Let them continue going on and on, and on, and on.

CPSIA information can be obtained
at www.ICGtesting.com
Printed in the USA
BVHW090927040222
627987BV00002B/37

9 781803 609904